ADVANCE PRAISE FOR
## Not Just a Pretty Face

This is a gripping, personal book by a recovered cosmetics addict with a great factual range on the impact of an unregulated group of companies, which have chemicalized the commercialization of beauty. This book should be read by women and men who have trusted, for too long, the companies whose products get inside their bodies and their minds, to the detriment of their health. Governments should require pre-market testing for safety. Ms. Malkan provides them with the evidence to finally act on behalf of consumers.

— Ralph Nader, consumer advocate, author of *Unsafe at Any Speed*

A must read for everyone. Writing this book at this time is most important. If we as a human race are not waking up to the realities within our biological systems, we humans are next on the endangered species list. Thank you Stacy for this most important investigation into the hidden dangers of everyday personal care

— Horst Rechelbacher, founder and former owner of Aveda

As a cancer survivor it is of great concern to me that the products I am using to make me beautiful on the outside are potentially making me ill on the inside. The skin is the largest organ in the body with the capability to absorb everything, so how is it possible that our skin products continue to go unregulated by the FDA? Shame on them for neglecting the American people in this way. Thank you Stacy for exposing the truth. The jig is up!

— Fran Drescher, New York Times best-selling author and star of the Emmy award-winning series *The Nanny*, visionary and president of the Cancer Schmancer Movement; uterine cancer survivor

As Stacy Malkan writes, the jars and bottles may be exquisite, but the truth is sadly painful about the ingredients in cosmetics and the defensiveness of the cosmetic industry. Her book is ⬚⬚⬚⬚⬚ and convincing call to women to take ⬚⬚⬚

they are exposing themselves and their unborn children to — and to do something about it. This book should be required reading for all teenagers, including the young men.

— Theo Colborn, PhD., leading scientist and expert on endocrine disruptors; president of TEDX (The Endocrine Disruptor Exchange); coauthor of *Our Stolen Future*

If you've ever thought twice about what's in your shampoo bottle or a tube of lipstick, it's thanks to the fine work of the Campaign for Safe Cosmetics. In *Not Just a Pretty Face*, Stacy Malkan introduces us to the brilliant and dedicated women behind the campaign, who have dared to take on Big Beauty and managed to reinvent the environmental movement at the same time. It's an inspiring and provocative take on an industry-gone-wild and what must be done to protect our health and the planet. Read this important book — you'll never look inside your bathroom cabinet in the same way again.

— Virginia Sole-Smith, environmental/women's health journalist

*Not Just a Pretty Face* underscores why we need Moms Rising, why we need a massive number of citizens' voices reminding our leaders about what their priorities need to be: safe products for our children and for ourselves. Together we can give our government a makeover.

— Joan Blades, cofounder of MoveOn.org and MomsRising.org; author of *The Motherhood Manifesto*

The jig is up for the cosmetic industry. Stacy Malkan's powerful compelling story of the overuse of unhealthy petroleum products in the stuff we put in our hair, on our face and over our body is so very important for us to hear, especially teenagers. She's clearly got the science down, but it is the fascinating stories of heroes and hope in the battle to "make over" the beauty industry that makes her book so readable.

— Don Hazen, executive editor, AlterNet.org

*Not Just a Pretty Face* is an entertaining and inspiring account of what we can all do to protect ourselves and our families from the toxic ingredients in our body care products and cosmetics.

The well-researched and dramatic stories of the scientists and activists who are working to protects us, their recent successes, and the tragedies that ensue because our government fails to regulate toxins are unforgettable. A must read for anyone who cares about our health and environment.

— Arlene Blum, PhD chemist; author of *Annapurna: A Woman's Place* and *Breaking Trail: A Climbing Life*

We are being exposed to toxins in personal care products without knowing it. *Not Just a Pretty Face* effectively conveys volumes of information while keeping us hanging page after page. Not only will you feel much more informed after you finish, you will also feel like you have just read a great mystery. Each and every American should read this book and take action.

— Sabrina McCormick, PhD; film director, *No Family History*, Robert Wood Johnson Health & Society Scholar, University of Pennsylvania

Crucial reading for anyone who has ever been to a drugstore. By examining advertising and the "beauty" industry, this book calls into question terms like "herbal" and "natural," and the very brands we have been taught to trust. Be prepared for the urge to take out and investigate every product in your bathroom cabinet.

— Jesse Epstein, documentary filmmaker, Wet Dreams and False Images (Distributed by New Day Films)

Stacy Malkan strips back the layers of the powerful cosmetic industry and reveals the truth about the personal care products we use daily. *Not Just a Pretty Face* offers up shocking information backed up by powerful studies and quotes from experts – all packaged in an accessible style that doesn't alarm but informs. What's more, Malkan provides to necessary tools to help consumers make better choices — for themselves, their children and the planet.

— Leslie Garrett, columnist and author of *The Virtuous Consumer: Your Shopping Guide for a Better, Kinder, Healthier World*

*For Carissa*

# Not Just a Pretty Face

## The Ugly Side of the Beauty Industry

Stacy Malkan

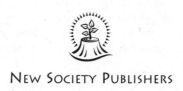

NEW SOCIETY PUBLISHERS

CATALOGING IN PUBLICATION DATA:
A catalog record for this publication is available from
the National Library of Canada.

Cover design by Diane McIntosh. Photo: iStock.

Printed in Canada.
Third printing October 2008.

Paperback ISBN: 978-0-86571-574-5

Inquiries regarding requests to reprint all or part of *Not Just a Pretty Face* should
be addressed to New Society Publishers at the address below. To order directly
from the publishers, please call toll-free (North America) 1-800-567-6772, or
order online at www.newsociety.com

Any other inquiries can be directed by mail to:

New Society Publishers
P.O. Box 189, Gabriola Island, BC V0R 1X0, Canada
(250) 247-9737

New Society Publishers' mission is to publish books that contribute in fundamental ways to building an ecologically sustainable and just society, and to do so with
the least possible impact on the environment, in a manner that models this vision.
We are committed to doing this not just through education, but through action.
This book is one step toward ending global deforestation and climate change. It is
printed on acid-free paper that is 100% post-consumer recycled (**100% old growth
forest-free**), processed chlorine free, and printed with vegetable-based, low-VOC
inks, with covers produced using Forest Stewardship Council-certified stock.
Additionally, New Society purchases carbon offsets annually, operating with a carbon-neutral footprint. For further information, or to browse our full list of books
and purchase securely, visit our website at: www.newsociety.com

NEW SOCIETY PUBLISHERS                                        www.newsociety.com

# Contents

# Acknowledgments

This book is a tribute to everyone who is working toward a healthier environment and a peaceful, just society. Special thanks to the former and current members and helpers of the Campaign for Safe Cosmetics, whose story I report in these pages. They include Charlotte Brody, Jane Houlihan, Bryony Schwan, Janet Nudelman, Jeanne Rizzo, Kevin Donegan, Marissa Walker, Lisa Archer, Andy Igrejas, Hema Subramanian, Lauren Sucher, Sean Gray, Cindy Luppi, Felicia Eaves, Mia Davis, Myriam Laura Beaulne, Genevieve Roja, Erin Johansen, Heather Sarantis, Esperanza Torres, Ann Blake, Susan Roll, Erin Boles, Dori Gilels, Alex Gorman, Erich Pica, Sabrina Williams and the folks at SmartMeme. Extra special thanks to Jane for your amazing research, Janet for meticulous record keeping, Kevin for co-leading the media efforts, Heather, Susan and Lee Kettleson for research that contributed to this book, and most especially Charlotte, my mentor and the inspirational force behind so many of the projects I've been fortunate to work on these past six years. A big thank-you to Gary Cohen, Anna Gilmore Hall and my colleagues at Health Care Without Harm for all your support, and to Peter Barnes and Mesa Refuge. Thanks to Dr. Ted Schettler, Nancy Evans and others who reviewed portions of this manuscript, to my kind and patient editor Betsy Nuse, to my boyfriend Jerry Caldwell, and to my support network of family and friends, especially

Kara, Kathy, Doug, Jami and my dads. From the bottom of my heart thank you to my mom, Diane Elizabeth Roche, for your endless encouragement and support, and for walking with me every step of the way. You are the best friend a girl could have, and I am truly blessed to have you in my life.

# *Prologue*

I confess: I've always been obsessed with cosmetics. When I was a *Seventeen*-magazine-reading high school cheerleader desperate to fit in, the Osco Drug cosmetics aisle was my comfort zone. With each measured purchase — cobalt blue eyeliner, soft rose blush — I was one step closer to that girl I dreamed of: the confident, lovable version of me. I spent hours in the bedroom with powders, puffs and that old familiar pink metal can of Aqua Net Extra Super Hold, spraying, spraying, spraying.

Years later, I left behind old Osco for the softly lit aisles of sultry Sephora, her $20 lip gloss seducing me to prove my worth. Heart racing, I toyed with the sparkling jars of Nars and MAC, playing math tricks in my head to figure out how I could possibly afford to stay loyal to the upper-end brand experience. These days, the pricey lip gloss lays gooey at the bottom of my bag. But just this morning, I lured myself out of bed with thoughts of orange sherbet shampoo and vanilla bean conditioner awaiting me in the hot shower.

Nowadays, my obsession is focused not so much on what beauty products can do to change me, but rather what I can do to change *them*. The cosmetics industry is in desperate need of a makeover. It is the unregulated, poorly studied chemical industry in a bottle. Toxic chemicals linked to cancer, birth defects and learning disabilities do not belong in products we smear on our bodies. Yet the world's richest cosmetics companies routinely use low levels of hazardous ingredients even though safer alternatives are available. "Why are they putting these toxic chemicals in cosmetics? One, because they can; two, because it's cheaper," Jared Blumenthal, director of the environment department for the City of San Francisco, explained to the crowd assembled in Union Square for "Project Prom."[1] The rally was organized by high school students who stood onstage alongside Blumenthal wearing prom dresses and combat boots to signify their war on toxic chemicals. "We are here to make a statement about our right to health," said high school junior Jessica Assaf. "We're here to say to the cosmetics industry, quit using crappy chemicals!" What an inspiring sight to behold: teenage girls aiming their combat boots at the billion-dollar beauty industry.

Our flashy beauty industry is a key supporting character in a drama that could be called "The Other Inconvenient Truth" — the messy problem that the material economy depends on toxic petrochemicals that are contaminating the human species and threatening our health. In Al Gore's famous movie "The Inconvenient Truth," the former US vice president warns that we must shift the economy to clean, renewable energy in order to avoid climate chaos. Similarly, we must also shift to non-toxic, non-polluting green chemistry technologies in order to protect our fertility and halt the growing epidemic of chronic diseases. Astonishingly, one in two men and one in three women are diagnosed with cancer in the United States, according to the National Cancer Institute. Asthma, autism, learning disabilities and infertility have all been rising. Replacing toxic chemicals with safer alternatives can reduce the number of people who develop these diseases.

The inconvenient truths of climate chaos and chemical contamination arise from the same mistake: our over-reliance on outdated, polluting technologies based on non-renewable fossil fuels. The problem of petroleum-derived chemicals is just much more personal — we're putting them on our faces and in our hair. Once you start asking questions about the products on the vanity table and under the bathroom sink it's hard to stop. You begin to see the world through new eyes. "The way we've been trained to perceive these things since we were young, it's all been subliminal. Whether it's 'hair so healthy it shines' — no, I'm sorry, not healthy; and herbal essences — no, not herbal. I had no idea until I got hold of this campaign," explained Kate Alver, a high school junior who volunteers with the Teen Campaign for Safe Cosmetics.

"I mean, you believe everything you hear, you believe everything you see, you think people are telling you the truth, you assume the best. You can't. You need to learn to train yourself to question things. And when you really go deep into the question, you find out so much more. And it's like a devastating effect, but obviously it's something you needed to find out. It's imperative for people to understand this."

This is a story about creating the world we want to live in. It's a story about the champions — the activists, moms, dads, scientists, politicians, workers, business owners, voters and smart shoppers — who are working toward a vision of a new green economy that is healthy for people and the environment. In the choices we make every day, starting with the products we put on our bodies, every single one of us can help turn that wheel of change.

Here's to our health, and to the children for seven generations to come.

Stacy Malkan
Berkeley, California
April 2007
www.NotJustaPrettyFace.org

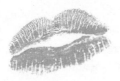

# 1

# *Indecent Exposure*

L ead in lipstick? We thought it was a hoax.

Even for watchdog environmentalists, those of us who monitor hazardous pollutants as part of our daily routines and read disturbing scientific data with our morning coffee, this one was a stretch. In recent years, researchers had found plenty of other toxic surprises lurking in the baby shampoo, men's cologne and various tubes of expensive makeup. But a heavy metal that reduces kids' IQs in products we're advised to "re-apply frequently" to the lips? An e-mail warning, circulating since 2003, had been widely dismissed. There was no time to follow the trail as the daily barrage of research, statistics and personal stories of the heart-rending kind sailed across our desks ...

## Baby Blues

The blood was quietly collected by the American Red Cross workers and sent to two independent laboratories to be analyzed for chemicals. The results were similar to previous studies: each person's body was contaminated with hundreds of industrial chemical compounds, including pesticides, stain repellents, flame retardants, plasticizers, even PCBs that were banned in the 1970s. But the subjects of this study were unlike any of the others. These were newborn babies, fresh from the womb.

The babies were born in US hospitals in August and September of 2004 and chosen at random by the Red Cross for the study conducted by the Environmental Working Group, a Washington DC research organization, and Commonweal, a California health and environmental group.[1] It was the first time such a wide range of pollutants had been measured in the umbilical cord blood of newborns who had never been in direct contact with industrialized society. The researchers detected a total of 287 chemicals in the babies' cord blood, including 180 chemicals that cause cancer in humans or animals, 217 that are toxic to the brain and nervous system, and 208 that cause birth defects or abnormal development in animal studies.

## Our Common Burden

Even if you have never marked an eyelash with mascara ... even if you are a Whole-Foods-shopping, careful consumer of all things "natural" ... even if you are a man (and after you read chapter 2, you might think *especially* if you are a man) ... this is your story. It's your story whether you live in New York City, the Arctic Circle or the top of the Rockies; no matter your race, nationality, age or income level.

It's your story and mine because all of us today share something unshared by countless generations of humans who lived before us: we carry man-made pollutants in our bodies. We inhale these toxicants from the air, drink them in our water, eat them in our food, spray them around our homes and rub them on our bodies. So it makes sense they'd also be in us. But only recently, with a scientific technique known as biomonitoring, have scientists been able to measure the actual levels of some synthetic chemicals that are getting into people — our so-called chemical body burden.

For several years, the US Centers for Disease Control and Prevention has been researching the body burden of thousands of average Americans. Government and independent researchers have studied human blood, urine and breast milk from

---

Daily Dose: How many personal care products did you use just this morning? Shampoo, deodorant, lotion, makeup — the average woman uses a dozen personal care products containing 168 chemical ingredients every day. Men use about six products a day containing 85 chemicals. We absorb, inhale and ingest many of these chemicals into our bodies.[2]

---

all regions of the world. The studies reveal that every single one of us is contaminated with scores of synthetic chemicals that are known to be toxic.[3]

So science now demonstrates what indigenous people have been saying all along: the environment is not out there, but *in here*. The same poisons running through the rivers are running through our veins.

## Intimate Details

Charlotte Brody was surprised by how she felt about her test results. "I wasn't one of these wavy gravy groovy people who didn't think I had chemicals in me," said the environmentalist and mother of two who was among the first people in the general population to be tested for a wide range of industrial chemicals.[4] "So I thought, I'll be the unemotional control person in the group." The tests revealed that Charlotte's body contained dioxin, PCBs, mercury, lead, cosmetic chemicals, lawn chemicals — 85 toxins in all — manufactured by companies such as Dow, Shell, Union Carbide, Exxon and Monsanto.

"I felt violated," Charlotte reported. She was especially upset about the pesticides. "I never used them in my house. They'd never been on my lawn. I bought organic whenever I could." Nevertheless, her body carried several variations of organophosphates and organochlorines that were designed to attack the nervous systems of insects. "How could Dow put Dursban into me when I never said they could — when I never used their product, never bought their product and never in my knowledge was in the presence of their product?" Charlotte wanted to know.

⚬──────⚬

Mary Brune remembers the exact moment she got angry. It was March 2005, and her baby Olivia had just turned six months old. "I came home one night after work and watched the TV news while nursing," Mary recalled. Texas Tech University had conducted a study of breast milk in 19 states and found that all the milk samples were contaminated with perchlorate, a component of rocket fuel.

"I'm sitting there on my couch nursing my daughter and I was stunned. I thought breast milk was as pure as it came as a food source for children. To find out there's all sorts of stuff in there: pesticides, mercury, lead … I was up all night thinking about it."

## Makeup Call

Michelle Hammond wasn't quite sure what to think. Hers was the first family in the United States to be biomonitored as part of a series of stories in the *Oakland Tribune*. "The results stunned even scientists," reported Douglas Fischer in the award-winning series.[5]

The tests found plasticizers, mercury, lead, cadmium and Teflon chemicals in the bodies of the two parents and two children. Five-year-old Mikaela had more dibutyl phthalate — a chemical used in cosmetics and other products — in her urine than 90% of kids tested in the US. But the biggest surprise was what they found in two-year-old Rowan: higher levels of flame retardant chemicals than had been found in nearly anyone else in the world — six times higher than the levels found in his parents, and twice the levels at which researchers start to see impaired fertility in male rats. "This is a very serious warning of very small children being heavily exposed," said Aake Bergman, professor of environmental chemistry at Stockholm University in Sweden, one of the world's foremost experts on human exposure to fire retardant chemicals.[6]

Nobody can say what effect, if any, the chemicals will have on the children's health. Biomonitoring studies detect chemicals in people at extremely low levels, but they can't predict health effects. However, the studies show that toxic chemicals are turning up where they shouldn't be, at the most precarious of times — in the sacred space of the womb and during the most at-risk times of childhood development.

"Parents know intuitively that babies in the womb are more vulnerable to the effects of industrial chemicals than adults," said Jane Houlihan, vice president of research at the Environmental Working Group and lead author of the cord-blood study. "This intuition is backed by science that has unfolded primarily over the past two decades."

Pound for pound, kids absorb more chemicals into their bodies, and their immature systems often don't detoxify and eliminate chemicals as efficiently as adults.[7] Studies show that even low doses of some chemicals — including ingredients found in everyday products such as baby bottles, furniture and cosmetics — can disrupt hormones, interfere with development and cause disease, particularly if exposures occur in the womb or early childhood.

In animal studies, the flame retardant chemicals found in Michelle Hammond's children — polybrominated diphenyl ethers (PBDEs) — can disrupt thyroid activity and harm brain development, while the cosmetic chemical dibutyl phthalate is toxic to the reproductive system, particularly for males. Yet very few studies had been conducted on humans, and there was no way to know for sure how these chemicals, or the many other toxins found in the kids, would impact their health.

Michelle had mixed emotions at her family's test results: she felt a bit angry and worried, but also empowered. "Yes of course I want to know what's in me and what's in my children. It was good to have information that was concrete," Michelle said. "OK so Rowan is high in PBDEs. What are they and how can I avoid them? What can I change to reduce my family's exposure to phthalates?" She set about trying to figure out where the exposures might be coming from.

Dibutyl phthalate seemed easier to avoid. Michelle knew the chemical was

"For years scientists have struggled to explain the rising rates of some cancers and childhood brain disorders. Something about modern living has driven a steady rise of certain maladies, from breast and prostate cancer to autism and learning disabilities. One suspect is now drawing intense scrutiny: the prevalence in the environment of certain industrial chemicals at extremely low levels. A growing body of animal research suggests to some scientists that even minute traces of some chemicals, always assumed to be biologically insignificant, can affect such processes and gene activation and the brain development of newborns.[8] "

— *Wall Street Journal,* Peter Waldman
"Common Industrial Chemicals in Tiny Doses Raise Health Issue"

used in cosmetics, and her daughter had recently taken a fancy to nail polish. "I'm not into makeup myself but I figured I'd let her play around with it if she wanted to," Michelle said. "It's fun. It's about playing with your identity ... But all of a sudden I started to wonder, what's in that makeup?" She'd read that some nail polish companies were removing dibutyl phthalate, so she went to the store and bought those less-toxic brands. The flame retardant chemicals were harder to pinpoint. "It felt impossible," Michelle said. So many products contain PBDEs, unlabeled and in unknown amounts — foam furniture, electronics, rugs, even clothing. Most consumer products are unregulated in the US, so manufacturers are allowed to use hazardous chemicals without demonstrating the safety of the products and without labeling them as toxic.

Now Michelle was starting to feel angrier. "Why do I have to worry about this? It just seems crazy that the government isn't more involved in making sure products are safe. I had no idea. So now I have to get involved." She traveled to Sacramento several times that year to testify before the California State Legislature, telling her family's story and advocating for bills to ban toxic chemicals. "I feel like I'm doing my small part," she said.

Her husband, Jeremiah Holland, suspects that the high levels of flame retardants found in his son aren't unusual. "What I believe is when you test more kids who are consistently putting their hands in their mouths ... you'll find that Rowan isn't abnormally high, but just one of all children being exposed to environmental pollutants at unprecedented levels."

## Our Chemical Legacy

Most of the synthetic chemicals found in the children didn't exist in the environment, never mind people's bodies, when my own grandmother Millie Pike Duggan was born in 1921. What an amazing changing century she witnessed! Life expectancy nearly doubled, the standard of living increased dramatically in some parts of the world, and human innovations changed the nature of the planet.

A major turning point came during World War II when government subsidies spurred the production of petroleum and its byproducts — the petrochemicals and plastics that would become the building blocks for the postwar material economy. Miracle makeup products, wrinkle-free clothes, stain-proof carpets, plastic toys and electronic gadgets galore now fill our homes and bring a wealth of convenience, fun and comfort to our lives. But there was an unforeseen dark side, as billions of tons of synthetic substances that never existed in nature before were released into the environment with little understanding about their impacts on the health of people and wildlife.

Then, as now, most chemicals were designed for function and efficiency, not health and safety. There was no cause-effect consciousness. A chemist might work to create a cheap polymer dye that was the perfect shade of crimson red, for instance, but he wasn't also making sure the dye was non-toxic, biodegradable and safe for children's health. Nobody was asking those questions. The government didn't require companies to ask those questions. Universities didn't require chemists to understand the biological and environmental impacts of the products they were creating. The majority of industrial chemicals were allowed onto the market with no safety testing to determine their health impacts.

Rachel Carson sounded an early warning about the chemical revolution and launched the modern environmental movement with her 1962 book *Silent Spring*.[9] The book revealed that the powerful pesticide DDT was not just killing insects, but irrevocably harming birds and wildlife and contaminating the entire world food supply. The chemical industry viciously attacked Carson, but her book held up to scientific scrutiny and led to the eventual ban of DDT in the US. A decade later, the human consequences of the chemical problem were broadcast to the world from the town of Love Canal, New York.

Lois Gibbs was living the typical American dream, except that her kids were sick. Since moving to Love Canal, her son had developed asthma and a urinary tract problem and her daughter was diagnosed with a rare blood disease. When Lois learned her son's school was built on a chemical waste dump, she tried to get him transferred but was told that would "set a bad precedent." So she started knocking on doors in her neighborhood with a petition to close down the school. After only a few blocks, it became apparent that the entire neighborhood was sick. Lois heard story after story of cancers, miscarriages and stillbirths. A formal health survey found a high percentage of birth defects in children born in the town. For three years, the families of Love Canal battled the chemical company that denied the problem and various government agencies that defended the company and refused to act, until finally, under pressure from media and the public, President Jimmy Carter signed a bill authorizing funding to permanently relocate the families. Congress later passed the Superfund law to clean up hazardous waste sites. "We stood together and demanded, demanded that the government make right," Lois said. "If a small community of working class families can bring the President of the United States to our stage, we can do anything if we stand together." [10]

Today, while some efforts have been made to reduce emissions and clean up hazardous waste sites, most chemicals in commerce are produced using the same outdated, polluting technologies developed decades ago. Every day, the US produces or imports 42 billion pounds of chemicals — enough to fill tanker trucks extending from San Francisco to Washington DC and back again. Over the next 25 years, global chemical production is expected to double in size, and the EPA predicts 600 new hazardous waste sites to appear each month in the US — adding to the 77,000 hazardous waste sites currently in the country.[11]

We may be living longer, but we're living sicker. Chronic diseases and disabilities now affect more than one third of the US population, according to the US Centers for Disease Control and Prevention.[12] Scientific studies have increasingly demonstrated that toxic chemicals are contributing to childhood cancer, hormone-related cancers, asthma, learning disabilities, birth defects, infertility and other health problems that have been increasing in recent decades.[13]

## Our Stolen Future

More than half of cosmetic products contain chemicals that can act like estrogen or disrupt hormones in the body, according to the 2005 *Skin Deep* report, an analysis of cosmetic ingredients conducted by the Environmental Working Group.[15]

Sterile bald eagles, alligators with small penises, panthers with abnormal testicles. In the 1996 book *Our Stolen Future,* zoologist Theo Colborn, PhD, documented countless reproductive and developmental disorders in wildlife and traced them back to synthetic chemicals that were interfering with the endocrine system, the body's main communication network that uses hormone messengers to regulate reproductive and developmental processes.[14] At low levels, some synthetic chemicals can mimic hormones in the body, acting like keys that turn receptor-mediated hormone functions on or off, thereby jamming up the message network. Such disruptions, the book reported, could profoundly impact intelligence, fertility and immune system functions — especially when exposures occurred during sensitive times of fetal development.

In the 10 years since the book's publication, Colborn and her co-authors have tracked the emerging science from animal studies, which continue to report that hormone-disrupting chemicals are harmful to development and reproduction. "There is an emerging pandemic of endocrine disorders in the Northern hemisphere," Colborn said at a recent conference about the links between chemical exposures and reproductive health and fertility.[16]

The evidence shows that:

- Chemical exposure can impact the hormonal system and disrupt normal development at doses far lower than previously suspected.[17]
- Genes and chemicals can work together to cause disease.[18]

- Mixtures of chemicals can have enhanced and unexpected health effects.[19]
- Early life exposures to synthetic chemicals can lead to health problems that don't show up until later in life (see "DES Story" below).

The new science calls into question the old way of thinking about chemical risk and disease — the idea that toxic chemicals cause some obvious health effect at some high dose, but lower doses are safe. This is the framework regulators use to calculate risk assessments and determine so-called tolerable intake levels of human exposure to hazardous chemicals. However, such risk assessments are likely to underestimate risk because they typically don't consider the sometimes surprising impacts of low-dose exposures, impacts on fetuses, chemical mixtures, interactions between genes and chemicals, or the broad range of health effects that can be caused by hormone disruption.

"Our health standards are in the Jurassic period," said Pete Myers, PhD, chief scientist of Environmental Health Sciences and co-author of *Our Stolen Future*. But Myers believes the emerging science carries an important silver lining.

Follow the latest scientific developments EnvironmentalHealthNews.org.

## DES Story

An intuitive mom first made the link: she asked her doctor if her use of diethylstilbestrol (DES) during pregnancy 20 years earlier could possibly have contributed to her daughter's vaginal cancer. The doctor didn't think so. But when another patient turned up in his office with the same rare type of cancer, the doctor thought to ask about DES use, and a case began to come together.

The pharmaceutical drug DES was a synthetic estrogen prescribed to millions of pregnant women in the US to prevent miscarriage. It was banned in 1971 after the discovery that "DES daughters" — daughters exposed to the drug in the womb — were developing cancer two decades after exposure. DES was also linked to higher rates of infertility, miscarriages and malformed reproductive tracts in the daughters. A study of DES daughters now over 40 found they are more than twice as likely to get breast cancer as women whose mothers did not take DES while pregnant.[20]

"It's telling us that a much larger proportion of the human burden of disease is preventable," Myers said. "I think that's really good news."

## The Poison Kiss

It turns out there is lead in lipstick, as two television reporters on opposite sides of North America reported in 2006. In July, Pittsburgh's WPXI-TV tested five brands of lipstick and found lead in every one of them. In May, Los Angeles' KCBS-TV tested 19 lip products and found lead in four of them, at levels that varied from 0.2 and 0.4 parts per million — that's two to four times the FDA limit for lead in candy.[21]

Is this trace level of lead cause for concern? It depends who you ask. For most healthy people, a little bit of lead in lipstick is "probably not a big deal, but there are people who need to be concerned about it and they are young women and pregnant women, for sure," said Devra Lee Davis, PhD, director of the Center for Environmental Oncology at the University of Pittsburgh Cancer Institute.[22] Lead builds up in the body, so small amounts applied to the lips several times daily, five days a week, could add up to a significant amount over a person's lifetime. Pregnant and nursing women pass lead and other hazardous chemicals on to their developing babies. Numerous studies show there is no safe dose of lead in children's blood.

None of this should worry the millions of women who enjoy lipstick every day, according to the cosmetics industry. As a Revlon representative explained in an e-mail to a concerned consumer named Emma Lougener:

---

*Dear Ms. Lougener:*

*We have received your comments and wish to thank you for taking the time to contact us. The following is a statement from the President of the Cosmetic, Toiletry, and Fragrance Association (CTFA):*

*"It is impossible to live in a lead-free world. Lead is ubiquitous in the environment. It is in the air, water, soil — in short it is unavoidable. Compared to the amount of lead a person would ingest from eating and drinking ordinary foods, the amount expected from the use of lipstick would be extremely small. In the US, the Food and*

*Drug Administration (FDA) has the responsibility to take action if it finds a product to be unsafe and has abundant legal authority to do so. Lipsticks are safe products that millions of consumers use and enjoy everyday. It is alarmist and irresponsible to suggest otherwise."*

*Thank you for your interest in Revlon products. We hope to continue serving your cosmetic needs.*

*Sincerely,*
*Rachel Evans*
*Sr. Consumer Services Representative*
*Revlon Consumer Information* [23]

---

It may be impossible to live in a lead-free world, but is it really impossible to keep lead out of lipstick? Aren't these the same companies with the glossy ads promising products that can bring balance, health and vitality to our lives? Shouldn't they be at the front of the line offering to reduce their contribution to the toxic load?

On the contrary, the world's richest cosmetics companies take the position that small amounts of hazardous chemicals are safe to use in cosmetics. The cosmetics industry's chief spokesperson, Dr. John Bailey, told the *New York Times* that the chemicals being singled out by environmental groups are present in such small amounts in personal care products that they pose no threat to human health. He compared them to salt in cooking. "A little salt on your peas or tomatoes can be good," Dr. Bailey said. "But a lot of salt can have adverse health effects on your blood pressure, and too much can be fatal."[24]

Unfortunately, mixtures of chemicals with various toxic properties become more complicated than salt. A little bit of hormone-disrupting chemicals mixed with carcinogenic contaminants in the baby shampoo, the bubble bath and the body wash add up — day in and day out. The cosmetics companies insist their products are safe, but what do those claims really mean? They typically mean the product has been tested to ensure it doesn't cause short-term obvious health effects, such as rashes, swelling and eye irritation. Most chemicals in cosmetics have not been tested for their potential to cause long-term health problems such as cancer or reproductive harm. Contrary to the letter from Revlon's Rachel Evans, the US FDA has little authority to ensure the safety of cosmetics or to remove unsafe products from the market. The way the system works in the US is that the cosmetics companies get to decide for themselves what's safe.[25] As you'll read in the pages ahead, companies are making decisions all over the board.

The cosmetics industry contributes more than just a little bit to the chemical problem. Hundreds of tons of chemical-containing beauty products are sold every day — and applied to people's bodies. According to a 1997 survey by the California Air Resources Board, more than 220 tons of personal care products were sold daily in the state, including 52 tons of hair spray, 24 tons of styling gels, 12 tons of fragrance and more — enough products to fill two tanker trucks per day with cosmetic chemical compounds, in just one state.[26]

## An Ounce of Prevention

If any of us went knocking on the neighbors' doors inquiring about health problems, what would we find? Who of us doesn't have a family member or close friend suffering from asthma, learning disabilities or cancer? One in eight American women is expected to get breast cancer in our lifetimes. My Nana Millie was one of those who did. Will I be one? Will you? What can we do?

Rather than waiting for the science to prove harm, industry and government must act on early warning signs of harm — an idea known as the precautionary principle. "If we're talking about the fact that what I'm eating and what products I'm using when I'm pregnant could affect my infant daughter's chance of developing breast cancer 40 years from now, how do you design a study to follow that? How do you fund a study like that? That's why we have to be precautionary," explained Brenda Salgado, program director of the advocacy group Breast Cancer Action. "If there's enough evidence from the lab and enough evidence from epidemiology that a substance can increase our risk of breast cancer, we have to be able to act on that, as a society, to reduce exposure. You're never going to have conclusive evidence of the kind that the chemical industries and current government system requires to prove that a chemical is causing breast cancer. It's not an isolated incident that happens in a vacuum. It just makes a lot more sense to act on early scientific warnings."

After lying awake all night thinking about the rocket fuel components in her breast milk, Mary Brune decided she needed to do something about it. She e-mailed the perchlorate story from the evening news to several of her friends who were new mothers and proposed they start an activist group. Not that any of them needed a new project. "Everyone was busy with new babies and starting back to work," Mary said. Nevertheless, "the response from everyone was an overwhelming yes. We all just recognized that it was something that needed attention." They named their new group MOMS for "Making Our Milk Safe." Now active in 37 states, MOMS advocates for government and corporate policies to eliminate harmful chemicals.[27]

"It distills down to moms taking back their bodies," Mary said. "This is an outrage that these toxic chemicals are allowed into the environment and end up in our bodies and our babies. We have to use our collective voting and purchasing power as moms to change it."

Women of all ages are likewise organizing to make change. As high school junior Sophie Lambert explained: "If we just get the word out and continue communicating with everyone, making changes — small changes and then increasingly larger changes — then we really can make a difference ... And soon, if we all just keep expanding our areas of where we're communicating, then eventually our campaign will just grow and maybe change the whole government around areas of health."

Good health begins with breastfeeding: Despite the presence of toxic chemicals in breast milk, experts agree that women should breastfeed their children. Breastfeeding provides significant health benefits to both mother and child. See lalecheleague.org. For more about MOMS, see safemilk.org.

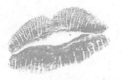

# 2

## *Not Too Pretty*

How could she write a report about nail polish? Jane Houlihan and Richard Wiles, two researchers at the Environmental Working Group, were having a debate. One of the top government watchdog groups in the US capital, EWG was busy writing exposes about dangerous pesticides in the country's food supply and tracking millions of dollars in wasteful subsidies to big agribusiness. Taking a few weeks out to write a report about nail polish seemed like a good way to get laughed out of the environmental community. But Jane Houlihan's discovery that a chemical linked to birth defects was a common ingredient in nail polish was unsettling. She suspected it wasn't the whole story either.

Besides getting dressed up for the occasional night out, Jane had never given much thought to cosmetics. As a civil engineer who spent ten years cleaning up toxic waste sites, she knew a lot about how chemicals move through the environment. And since having two kids, she had a keen interest in children's health. In her mid 30s, Jane merged her interests into a new career as vice president of research at the Environmental Working Group, specializing in exposing the health risks from toxins in food, air, water and consumer products. But she never wove together the threads of cosmetics, chemicals and children's health until a warm day in October 2000.

The US Centers for Disease Control had just released new research from their study of the levels of toxic chemicals in the bodies of average

Americans. The CDC scientists found seven different types of phthalates — a set of industrial chemicals linked to birth defects in the male reproductive system — in 289 people tested. Every single person had dibutyl phthalate (DBP), the most toxic of the phthalates, in his or her body. The ubiquity of phthalates in the general population surprised the scientists. "From a public health perspective, these data provide evidence that phthalate exposure is both higher and more common than previously suspected," they wrote.[1]

But the biggest surprise came when they broke down the data by age and gender. In their paper, the CDC researchers reported that women age 20 to 40 appeared to have the highest levels of DBP in their bodies. This was a concern. Women in this group — childbearing age — were the ones who would be most likely to expose their developing babies to DBP, a chemical that causes birth defects and lifelong reproductive problems in male animals exposed in the womb.[2] Where were the women's exposures coming from? The CDC scientists didn't know. But in their paper they speculated on many possible sources, including a wide range of cosmetics and personal care products.

"As soon as I read that, I thought wow. Here's this chemical, a potent reproductive toxicant, in our bodies, and it's possibly because of cosmetics," Jane Houlihan said. She knew cosmetics had labels on the back, even though she'd hardly bothered to read them because they're so difficult to interpret. So she decided to do a little detective work. She headed across the street to the Rite Aid in Dupont Circle and started reading labels. "I looked for phthalates, looked for phthalates, looked for phthalates," up and down the shampoo section, deodorant, face cream and makeup sections. She went cross-eyed trying to make out tiny words on nail polish bottles. There, she found what she was looking for. More than half the nail polishes had the phthalate DBP listed on the labels.

Jane went back to the office with some samples of DBP-containing nail polish and a big question: The CDC researchers had said in their paper that phthalates were in a wide range of cosmetics; why was she finding them only in nail polish? It was the right question for the right person. Jane had great patience — a love even — for meticulous research. In college, she had switched her major from piano to civil engineering because she "missed math and science too much." Now that she was intrigued by the data about phthalates in cosmetics, she was determined to follow the trail. She found more clues sifting through the US patent database, searching for sample product formulations. Sure enough, phthalates were proposed for a wide range of cosmetic products. Jane documented all the patents she could find.

## Maybe He's Born with It, Maybe It's ...

Phthalates is not the most convenient word to work with — weird to spell and hard to figure out how to pronounce (THA-lates). But the chemicals have an important story to tell about the science and politics of chemicals. You may be surprised to learn you are already intimately familiar with phthalates: think of the potent aroma of a vinyl shower curtain or "new car smell." Produced in the amount of one billion tons per year worldwide, phthalates are used to soften vinyl plastic and hold scent and color in a variety of consumer products. More than two decades ago, scientists began building a body of evidence that phthalates can be powerful reproductive and developmental toxicants in laboratory animals, particularly for males exposed in the womb.

"For 25 years we've known that phthalates disrupt the production of testosterone critical for the masculinization of the male species," said Earl Gray, a top phthalate researcher at the US Environmental Protection Agency.[3] Hundreds of animal studies show that phthalates like dibutyl phthalate (DBP) can block male hormones called androgens, which are responsible for making a male into a male. The result of this anti-androgen effect is what scientists call "de-masculinization" of male offspring: low sperm counts, testicular atrophy, undescended testicles and birth defects of the penis such as hypospadias, where the opening of the urethra occurs on the underside of the penis instead of the tip. This spectrum of health effects is so common in lab animals exposed to phthalates that scientists have come to call it "phthalates syndrome."

But what does that mean for people? Limited human data was available. The method to detect phthalate metabolites in human fluids had only recently been developed by CDC scientists John Brock and Benjamin Blount and reported in their October 2000 paper. Human health trends over the past few decades provided a possible clue. A similar spectrum of health effects found in the lab animals exposed to certain phthalates was also occurring in people: sperm counts appeared to be declining in industrialized countries, birth defects of the male reproductive tract had been increasing, and testicular cancer was on the rise. Scientists called these human health effects "testicular dysgenesis syndrome," and some suspected the disorders could be caused by phthalates and other chemicals that interfere with male sex hormones. But a cause and effect relationship had not been established definitively; there was no proof phthalates were harming people — just new evidence that phthalates appeared to be getting into everyone's bodies.

## Beauty Secrets

Charlotte Brody was driving her sons crazy with the label reading. "We couldn't just go to the grocery store," said the registered nurse and mother of two. "I'd think of a new product group. Oh, we haven't looked at hair mousses, so we'd go read the labels of all the mousses in the store." Like Jane, Charlotte was looking for phthalates. It was a subject close to her heart. Besides knowing her own body burden load of the chemicals — three different types of phthalates were in her body at the time of her biomonitoring test — she had been following the science on phthalates for years in her job as executive director of Health Care Without Harm, an international coalition that works on reducing the environmental impact of the health care industry.

The group was founded in 1996 after the US Environmental Protection Agency named medical waste incinerators as the leading source of dioxin, one of the most potent carcinogens. Health Care Without Harm was pushing hospitals to phase out medical devices made of vinyl plastic, which created dioxin when manufactured and burned, and which also had a second problem: they leached phthalates into patients. Vinyl medical devices such as IV bags were softened with di-2-ethylhexyl phthalate (DEHP), a close cousin of the phthalate Jane found in the nail polish. The same month the CDC released its findings about phthalates in people, an expert panel at the US National Toxicology Program expressed "serious concern" that phthalates leaching from vinyl medical devices could harm the reproductive organs of critically ill male infants receiving medical treatments. The NTP scientists said the animal studies on phthalates were likely to predict human health impacts, and they were concerned that healthy male fetuses and infants could be harmed if they were exposed to phthalates by non-medical sources while in the womb or during the first years of life.[4]

If cosmetics were a source of phthalates, that could mean potentially high exposures to pregnant women and babies in the womb. But Charlotte and her sons had done an exhaustive label search of cosmetics during their trips to the grocery store, and found no phthalates except in the nail polish.

Meanwhile, Jane Houlihan and Richard Wiles were down the street at the Environmental Working Group deciding whether to write the report about nail polish and risk getting laughed out of the environmental community. Jane decided to give it a shot. Through label searches, she found the phthalate DBP in 37 popular nail polishes, top coats and hardeners made by L'Oréal, Maybelline, Oil of Olay and Cover Girl among other popular brands. In her searches at the US patent office, she found patents proposing to use phthalates in a broad range of cosmetic products, from shampoos to deodorant — even gum, candy and pharmaceutical drugs. Procter & Gamble had the highest number, 37 out of the 100 patents she analyzed.

Jane wrote up the results in a report she called *Beauty Secrets: Does a Common Chemical in Nail Polish Pose Risks to Human Health?* [5] "We purposefully phrased the subtitle of the report as a question," Jane explained. "Clearly you don't want to come out of the box saying your nail polish is killing you, when that's not at all where the evidence is. So we just raised a lot of questions in that report. We asked if nail polish is a big source of dibutyl phthalate in people. And we said that we don't know."

Nobody knew, Jane said, because nobody was looking. Nobody had tested nail salon workers to see if they had high levels of DBP in their bodies. Nobody had tested the air in nail salons to see if it contained high levels of the toxic chemical. Nobody was looking for patterns of disease among nail salon workers or their babies. In addition to the huge gaps in health research, *Beauty Secrets* documented major loopholes in federal law that allow companies to put unlimited amounts of toxic and untested chemicals into products. "Contrary to popular belief, industrial chemicals in consumer products are essentially unregulated in the United States," Jane reported. "Except for chemicals added directly to food, there is no legal requirement for health and safety testing or human exposure monitoring for any chemical in commerce." [6] *Beauty Secrets* was released at the National Press Club in Washington DC on November 28, 2000. With the nation focused on a still-undecided election, it was a quiet day for news at the Press Club, though some reporters — mostly female — showed up for the event.

Charlotte Brody was there, sitting in the back row bouncing her high-heeled boot, feeling anxious. "I'm sitting there looking at the hands of all the women in the room, and I thought: I just don't buy it. I don't buy that the main source of phthalates in personal care products is nail polish," she recalled. "It wouldn't be enough to explain the difference of why CDC found more phthalates in women." Another small study had caught Charlotte's attention: Jane Hoppin at the National Institutes of Environmental Health Sciences reported that African-American women in the Washington DC area had twice the levels of DBP in their bodies as the general population. "Where was it coming from? We knew that there were phthalates in food wraps and food containers, vinyl shower curtains, vinyl flooring and wall coverings. But why would there be a difference in gender? Why would there be a difference in African Americans? Something else was going on."

Charlotte wasn't going to let it go. After three decades of activism, including running a group of Planned Parenthood clinics in the South in the 1980s, she had developed quite a bulldog determination. It mixed well with Jane's tenacity for the details. Together, they hatched a plan: they would purchase a range of beauty products and send them to an independent laboratory to test for phthalates. "First we batch tested," Charlotte explained. "We would buy African-American hair products, take a tiny bit of each, stir them together and test that mixture, because we didn't have much money. Eventually we figured out that we wanted to test products that were most in use. So we found our way to the chain drugstore weekly, which publishes a report every year of the most popular brands. We bought those brands in the product categories that batch tested positive." They chose 72 products and sent them off to an independent laboratory in Chicago.

## Organizing Like a Girl

Bryony Schwan, the founder of Women's Voices for the Earth, was skeptical when Charlotte asked her to help with the project. Cosmetics? "As a feminist, initially it was hard for me to think about cosmetics when certain communities were suffering so much from pollution," Bryony said. She was all too familiar with the plight of environmentally devastated communities in Montana, where the rivers run red with toxic mining waste. In the early 1990s, Bryony worked for a conservation organization on protecting endangered species habitats. Through that experience, she also became all too familiar with the male-dominated culture of environmental organizing. There were hardly any female leaders in the work, even though women from polluted communities seemed to be the ones who had the most passion for the issues. "I would see women come to meetings and get engaged but they wouldn't stay engaged," Bryony said. "They would be very concerned and they would say, 'What can we do?' and some guy would turn around and say, 'Why don't you bring tea and cookies to the next meeting?' Seriously, I'm not making it up."

Meetings were aggressive, table-thumping affairs with frequent sports and war terminology and it was hard to get a word in edgewise. Many women stopped coming after their first or second time. Bryony remembers one meeting that erupted into a shouting match over who could call a certain member of the US Congress the worst name in the loudest voice. The women at the table, one by one, got up to leave. They were gathered in the next room standing near the copy machine, discussing their desire to have a more productive work environment, when one of the men came out of the room holding a stack of papers. He asked the women if they could please make him some copies.

Bryony decided to try a different way. She organized a women's-only environmental conference in the fall of 1994, and more than 100 women from across the Northern Rockies — who "all told stories like that" — came out for the event. The enthusiasm for a women's organizing vehicle convinced Bryony to launch Women's Voices for the Earth in 1995 with $11,000 in operating money. It was tough going at first. "Funders would look at me funny and say, 'I don't get it. Why a women's group? Why are you separating them out?'" The answer was that she felt strongly that the environmental debate needed to focus on women, with women taking the lead.

"Women are the canaries in the coal mine in a lot of ways. By biology and for other reasons, we are disproportionately impacted by environmental pollution," she said. As the ones who bear children, breast feed, live in greater numbers in low-income polluted communities and deal more directly with sick kids and relatives, women have more first-hand experience with the health consequences of toxic pollution. As the primary buyers of household goods and the largest voting block in the US, women also have the power to change the situation by demanding better laws and safer products. "There is so much untapped potential in women. We haven't been engaged in high-level decision making and we need to be. Our health is not protected," said Bryony.

She also felt that, in order to engage women, the environmental debate needed to focus on issues relevant to the everyday lives of families. For that reason, she finally came around on the cosmetics question. "I realized that while people are sympathetic about the situation in the fence-line communities, while they feel bad about it, it's not their situation. It's happening to somebody else. I started to think that cosmetics were a good way to tell the story that this is happening to everybody. It's personal. It's not pollution coming out of a smokestack; we're putting this stuff on our own bodies," she explained. "We're being told that we're using these products to help our health and beauty and, quite frankly, it's the opposite." Women's Voices for the Earth joined Health Care Without Harm and the Environmental Working Group in writing a report about the lab results from Chicago.

## Late Nights and Sticky Notes

Preliminary results from the lab indicated there would be interesting news to share, and the fundraising had gone well. A donor agreed to put up money for a full-page ad in the *New York Times*. Now there were partners across the country: ad designers in San Francisco, science advisors in Boston and Michigan, Jane writing the report in DC in perfectionist detail as she did everything, with the help of Bryony in Montana. Charlotte was in the apartment-sized DC offices of Health Care Without Harm trying to keep the train on the track. The report writing was going painstakingly slowly. The final lab results were delayed, and delayed again. If anyone could keep the project going, it was Charlotte. In her years of organizing, she had forged winning coalitions among diverse interests — nuns, nurses, activists and hospital executives, for example. The secret, she said, is "organizing like a girl."

"Relationships matter," Charlotte said. Organizing like a girl, in her words, means that "winning today's argument but losing a long-term ally is not a good deal. That you recognize that you like some people better than other people, but you don't confuse who you like best with what coalition partners you need to win. And most importantly, that if you're worrying about who gets the credit and if your face got the most seconds on television, you're not worrying about the right thing — how much progressive social change can we win in any situation. It's a girl thing, to watch what you've helped do invisibly become visible, and to be happy to have been of service to the universe."

It wasn't always easy to work with many cooks in the kitchen, though, especially with the deadline pressure on. Tensions were rising. Charlotte could also be fierce. I was trying to help hold things together in my role as communications director of Health Care Without Harm. One night after everyone else had gone home, Charlotte and I sat at the conference table in the front office with pads of colored sticky notes. We wrote down each task that had to be done, one task per sticky note, until the table was covered end to end with colored squares. We stared at the squares, feeling solemn. Who thought this project was a good idea? We divvied up the squares and headed home. It was tempting to stay there.

## Not Too Pretty

"July 10, 2002 — New product tests find unlabeled toxin in many best selling cosmetics," announced the press release. The lab had found phthalates in nearly three quarters of the 72 products tested — popular brands of hair spray, deodorant, hair gel, body lotions and every single fragrance tested. Brands included Cover Girl, Pantene, Secret and Vidal Sassoon (by Procter & Gamble); Dove, Escape, Eternity, Suave and Salon Selectives (by Unilever); Clairol, L'Oréal and Revlon. None of the products had the word "phthalates" listed on the label.[7]

My favorite product from the old days, Aqua Net Professional Hair Spray, contained more than one phthalate, as did Healing Garden Pure Joy Body Treatment, Secret Sheer Dry Regular deodorant and Revlon's Fire and Ice Cologne Spray. But the worst offender — it was hard to believe — was Poison perfume. The aptly named fragrance made by Christian Dior contained four different types of phthalates.

Poison was the product the ad designers chose to highlight in a full-page ad in the *New York Times*. "Sexy for her. For baby, it could really be poison," said the headline over the full-page photo of a pretty young pregnant woman sniffing a bottle of perfume. The *Times* insisted on air-brushing the product name off the photo, but many women nevertheless recognized the contoured shape of the Poison bottle. The ad listed the names of all the phthalate-containing products. It ran the same day the press conference was scheduled to take place at Washington DC's National Press Club.

"Major loopholes in federal law allow the $20-billion-a-year cosmetics industry to put unlimited amounts of phthalates into many personal care products with no required testing, no required monitoring of health effects, and no required labeling," said the *Not Too Pretty* report.[8] "To our knowledge, the 72 products detailed in this study represent the most comprehensive information available on the occurrence of phthalates in individual beauty care products." Yet the study represented just a tiny fraction of products on the market. And because phthalates weren't listed on the labels — due to a huge loophole that allows companies to keep the ingredients in fragrance a secret — there was no way for consumers to tell which brands had the chemicals in them. "We spent $175 per product to determine if phthalates are present, a cost hardly within the budget of most pregnant women trying to steer clear of myriad products that could potentially harm a fetus," the report said.

Jane, Charlotte and Bryony arrived early to the Press Club and waited nervously in the empty Murrow Room. After all that drama, would anyone even show up? The boys from the Environmental Working Group arrived first and filed into the front row. There was a something-to-prove feeling in the air. This was, after all, the girls' project. About cosmetics. At about quarter to the hour, reporters started filing in until every seat in the house was taken and the back of the room was packed with cameras. That night, and over the next few weeks, the story of phthalates in cosmetics aired on more than 600 television news stations across the US. The toxic danger lurking in their shampoo was suddenly on the minds of Americans from coast to coast.

## Europe's Fashion Sense

Helena Norin was flipping through newspapers in her office in Stockholm, Sweden, on a cold November day. She could hardly believe her eyes. The story about phthalates in cosmetics was in every major newspaper in the country, and all over the radio and TV. In 30 years of environmental organizing, the Swedish Society for Nature Conservation had never seen so much press coverage of one of their issues. They had just released their new report *Pretty Nasty,* a European version of the *Not Too Pretty* report. Similar to what the US groups had done, Norin and her collaborators at Women's Environmental Network in the UK and Health Care Without Harm Europe had bought beauty products from stores in Britain and Sweden and sent them to a lab to test for phthalates.

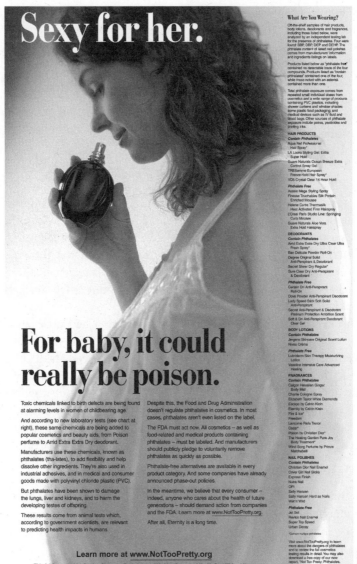

This full-page ad ran in the New York Times *with the release of the* Not Too Pretty *report, which found that 72% of products tested contain phthalates, a chemical linked to birth defects. The ad named all phthalate-containing products and featured Poison perfume, the product that contained the most phthalates — four different types.*

The European results were similar to the American: 79% of products — popular deodorants, perfumes, hair sprays, mousses and gels — contained phthalates, and more than half contained multiple phthalates.[9] The story got more attention than anyone could remember "because these are products that people use every day, products that people put on our own bodies," Helena suspected. "When you are a Swede buying something in Sweden, you think someone has checked this product and it must be safe to use." But the revelation that most products contained phthalates hit a nerve in her country. "Many people got quite frustrated. They thought someone took care of this for them. But we had to tell them this is not the case. You have to check for yourself." But that was the most frustrating part. "A lot of people were asking what to do, but it's hard to give advice. What do you tell people?" As in the US, the European environmental groups could test only a small number of products, leaving an open question as to which of the thousands of other products on store shelves contained phthalates. As in the US, it was legal for companies to put unlimited amounts of phthalates and other toxic chemicals into cosmetic products.

But in Europe, that was just about to change. The European Union (EU) was getting ready to pass a new amendment to the Cosmetics Directive, the law that regulates cosmetics in all EU countries (15 countries at the time). The new amendment would ban animal testing of cosmetics, which was getting a lot of press attention, but it would also do something else that had slipped under the media radar: it would ban chemicals that were known or highly suspected of causing cancer, birth defects or genetic mutation from use in cosmetics. Two phthalates, DEHP and DBP, were on the prohibited list, along with hundreds of other chemicals. The phthalates were classified as Class 2 reproductive toxicants in the EU, meaning they were highly suspected of causing reproductive damage.[10] The new Cosmetics Directive was a major regulatory shift, one that could have huge implications for the cosmetics industry.

## Fox Guards the Henhouse

Most people in the US believe the government makes sure personal care products are safe. However, this is not the case. The US Food and Drug Administration does not have the authority to require companies to safety test personal care products before they go on the market and cannot even recall defective or possibly harmful cosmetics. Instead, the industry gets to "police itself" through a group called the Cosmetic Ingredient Review (CIR) panel. The CIR panel is funded and run by the cosmetics industry through its trade association, the Cosmetic, Toiletry, and Fragrance Association. The panel has seven voting members, with non-voting memberships for the trade association, the FDA and a consumer group.

Charlotte and Jane were about to get a good look at how this system works. On November 19, 2000 — four months after the *Not Too Pretty* report made national headlines in the US and just one week after the European governments reached agreement to ban two phthalates from cosmetics — the CIR panel was scheduled to debate the science on phthalates. Jane and Charlotte had sent extensive written comments to the panel about the *Not Too Pretty* report findings, and they were invited to testify at the panel's meeting at the Monarch Hotel in downtown Washington DC.

From the start, the CIR panel meeting had disturbing dynamics. The first thing Jane noticed is that the panel was dominated by dermatologists who, for a living, think about allergies and skin sensitizers. They didn't have the experience or expertise to evaluate risks to the reproductive system of chronic exposure to phthalates over time. They also had little information about how much people are being exposed to phthalates from cosmetics. For their review of dibutyl phthalate, the panel relied on penetration studies in cadaver skin (dead people) to figure out how much phthalates might be getting into people from cosmetics, and they didn't consider exposures in enclosed, heavy-use areas such as nail salons. They also relied on the "safe level" of exposure set in the 1990s by the Environmental Protection Agency, which was derived from a 1953 study that didn't look at the reproductive effects of phthalates. Besides all that, Jane noticed early on in the deliberations that the panel was being heavily influenced by cosmetics industry representatives. At one point when a question arose from the panel about exposure levels, Gerald McEwan, the vice president of science at the trade association, "was literally calculating exposure numbers on, basically, his lunch napkin and then feeding those numbers to the panel," Jane said.

Charlotte Brody was the one to explain the European Union plan to ban chemicals suspected of causing cancer and birth defects from cosmetics. "There seemed to be real surprise in the room when I talked about the EU ban," she recalled. Eyes turned to Gerald McEwan of the trade association, "and he said it wasn't true. He said that maybe there was some kind of proposal, something Greenpeace was proposing in Europe, but it wasn't about to become law. I said to them, you don't have to take my word for it, call the European Union. Why would I lie about what the European Union was going to do?"

McEwan later told a reporter he was surprised by the EU decision to ban chemicals from cosmetics, and that companies in Europe were doing what they could to influence the situation. If the new EU directive went forward as written, he said, it would have limited short-term impacts on the cosmetics industry, causing the removal of a few ingredients. But over the long term, it could have profound consequences on the industry, he said, since the ban applied not only to chemicals currently on the banned blacklist, but to all chemicals added in the future.[11]

Despite the industry lobbying efforts, the EU approved the new Cosmetics Directive as written. But in the US, it was obvious the cosmetics industry held more sway. After about an hour of debate, the CIR panel issued its ruling that phthalates were "safe as currently used" in cosmetics. "We laid out all of the science on phthalates for them and they essentially said that, yes, phthalates can be dangerous, but not at the low levels present in cosmetics," Charlotte explained. "I didn't expect them to ban phthalates. But I expected them to say less is better than more, and we need the industry to produce more data, and it would be good if there wasn't exposure to pregnant women from these products." But "safe as currently used" was the end of the story as far as the US government was concerned, thanks to the authority of the Cosmetic Ingredient Review panel. The girls would have to organize another way.

## Boys Will be Boys ... or Will They?

By the summer of 2005, phthalates were all over the news again, due to a first-of-its-kind human study by Shanna Swan, PhD, professor of obstetrics and gynecology at the University of Rochester. Swan measured the levels of phthalates in the bodies of pregnant women, then studied their male infants after birth. The study found "a significant relationship" between the levels of phthalates in the mothers' bodies during pregnancy and changes in the genitals of their baby boys.[12] The pregnant women with the highest phthalate levels — equivalent to the levels currently found in about a quarter of US women — were more likely to have baby sons with smaller penises and incompletely descended testicles. The boys were also more likely to have a shorter distance from their anus to their penis (called anogenital distance, or AGD), which is an indicator of masculinity. The distance is about half as long in girls as it is in boys. "None of our boys looked weird; they weren't grossly deformed," Swan explained. "But they had subtle differences."

The chemical industry was quick to criticize the study, saying it was small and flawed. "There is no reliable evidence that any phthalate, used as intended, has ever caused a health problem for a human," said Marian Stanley of the Phthalates Ester Panel, the trade group that promotes and defends phthalates.[13] Swan conceded the study was small and needs to be repeated. She planned to do a larger follow-up study, and to follow the boys in the original study to see if their play behaviors tend toward feminized play patterns.

In addition to Swan's study, other human studies on phthalates had started to emerge. Harvard School of Public Health researchers Dr. Russ Hauser and Susan Duty studied men in an infertility clinic and found that men who had higher levels of DBP in their bodies had lower sperm quality and lower sperm motility.[14] In a separate study of 379 men from an infertility clinic, the Harvard researchers correlated diethyl phthalate (DEP) with DNA damage in the men's sperm, a condition that can lead to infertility or miscarriage.[15] DEP is the phthalate used most widely in cosmetics. The chemical appears to be getting into people's bodies from the products, according to another study conducted by Dr. Hauser's team. Men who used cologne or aftershave within 48 hours before urine collection had more than twice the levels of DEP in their bodies as men who did not use cologne or aftershave, the study found. For each additional type of personal care product used, the DEP metabolite in their bodies increased by 33%.[16]

## Take Charge of Your Health

The decades of animal research and emerging human studies indicated phthalates may be a problem for male reproductive health — but still there was no proof. "The data are starting to suggest that there may be a potential risk" to humans from phthalates, said Dr. Russ Hauser from the Harvard School of Public Health, who describes himself as cautious in interpreting the data. Though phthalates have been well studied in animals, the human data is new and limited and has involved small populations, he said.

The research is challenging. There are at least ten different types of phthalates, and they are typically studied one at a time. Though preliminary

## A Mother's Story

Olivia James first heard about phthalates from her sister Karen Johnson, executive vice president of the National Organization for Women. Karen had spoken at the press conference organized by environmental groups after the CIR panel exonerated phthalates. She had come to make a general statement about women's right to know about toxic exposures. But after hearing the science presentations, Karen added a personal story to her speech: her sister Olivia, a former fashion model, had given birth to a premature son with a birth defect of the penis. She wondered if phthalates and cosmetics could be connected.

Olivia got the phone call from Karen right afterward. "She said you need to check this out," recalled Olivia. "This could be what happened with DJ. So I looked into it. I started reading articles about phthalates and looking it up on the Web." Olivia had a lot of questions. She wanted to ask her old doctor if he thought phthalates could be connected to her son's birth defect, but he had long since retired.

For 16 years, Olivia had worked as a runway model. She spent hours getting made up for shoots, using dozens of products, including full body makeup. Even when she wasn't working, she covered herself in the products of her clients and wore top-notch makeup each time she went out the door because "you just never know." After her September 1994 wedding, Olivia stopped modeling. "I was tired. I wanted to give my marriage a chance. I wanted to start a new chapter," she said. And she really wanted a baby. After one miscarriage, she was thrilled beyond belief when she got pregnant with DJ in 1996.

During her pregnancy, Olivia was "still in that model frame of mind. I never wanted to be the typical pregnant woman you see out there with old house shoes on, looking tired, with stretchy pants on and the same sweater every day." So she colored her hair and made frequent trips to the nail salon — at least once a week to get her nail tips touched up, sometimes twice a week ☛

evidence suggests that the effects of the chemicals are cumulative — with combined phthalates having greater health effects than any one acting alone — researchers have struggled with how to quantify that. "Everyone's thinking about the need to study mixtures," Dr. Hauser explained, "but the question of how to do it is what's difficult. It's

to get the colors changed on her fingers and toes for five bucks a pop. One week she went to the nail salon every day.

DJ was born 10 weeks early in February 1997. "He was so early, I was afraid to attach myself to him," Olivia recalled. "It was really hard, we wouldn't make plans, we didn't think he was going to make it." At six weeks, when he was three pounds ten ounces, DJ was finally allowed to go home, but he needed surgery to correct a birth defect of the penis called hypospadias, in order to bring the opening of the urethra in line with the end of the penis. The condition was common with premature babies, the doctor told Olivia, and they didn't know why it happened. DJ's case was severe, he said, but not as severe as some cases he'd seen.

DJ had the surgery just before Thanksgiving at the age of eight months. The next couple of weeks were rough. "What was hard, I always knew when he wet his diaper, he was so raw … he would scream and cry in pain because it would burn," Olivia recalled. "It was really hard to deal with. Babies don't understand. You can't comfort them. There's nothing you can do. That's something I would never want anyone to have to go through."

DJ healed up and is fine today, with no noticeable scar from the surgery. And the boy who was once so small now looks big for his age. At 106 pounds, he is 5 feet tall and wearing a man's size 10½ shoe at the age of 9. "The doctor said at this rate he's predicting 6 feet 4," Olivia says proudly. The model glamour still shines in her smile as Olivia talks about DJ, her obvious pride and joy. She'll always wonder if phthalates were connected to his health problems, but she knows she'll never know for sure. She tells his story because she thinks it's important for the information to get out to women. "DJ knows all about it and he knows what I'm doing [telling his story] and he's not embarrassed by it. He agrees people should know," Olivia said. Her feeling is that if there's suspicion around phthalates, the cosmetics companies should just stop using the chemicals. "Does it cost them a lot to reformulate? No, because they've had to do it for Europe anyway. Then, duh, wouldn't you want to do it here?"

extremely important and hopefully we'll make some progress in that area." He also noted that people are "exposed to not only phthalates but hundreds of other chemicals," including others that block the male androgen hormone as phthalates appear to do. How can researchers quantify those mixtures? One thing Dr. Hauser was sure of regarding phthalates: "In the next two to three years, there will be quite a bit of new research coming out, including on females," he said. "In the next few years there should be more data and confirmatory studies."

Will we ever know for certain if phthalates are harming people? Due to the limitations of the science, proof may not be possible. Do we know enough to act? Dr. Shanna Swan thinks so. "The risks [of phthalates], while not established conclusively, are very probable to humans, and the benefits are not clear to me," Swan said when she testified at a California legislative hearing in favor of a bill to ban phthalates from toys.[17] "These chemicals are hardly essential — in most cases, safer alternatives do exist," Swan wrote in the *San Francisco Chronicle*. "California would do well to ban these toxins from the products to which children are regularly exposed. In the meantime, however, parents can take steps of their own."[18]

The European Union, using a precautionary approach, has already banned certain phthalates from children's toys, as well as cosmetics. But in the US, consumer products can contain unlimited amounts of phthalates and most other hazardous chemicals. And even though toy manufacturers are already making phthalate-free toys for Europe, toys sold in the US still contain the chemicals, according to product tests conducted by the *San Francisco Chronicle* in 2006. The tests found phthalates in a baby's teething ring made by Prestige Brands, a Goldberger's Fuzzy Fleece Baby doll and a yellow rubber ducky sold at Walgreens.[19] In the absence of federal leadership, some US states are acting on their own. California, New York and Maryland introduced legislation to ban phthalates from toys or cosmetics in the 2004–2006 legislative sessions. The chemical industry lobbied extensively against the bills, and none passed. But the push for protective laws continues. In 2006, the city of San Francisco banned several phthalates, as well as the hormone-disrupting chemical bisphenol A, from children's toys. The city was subsequently sued by the chemical industry trade association. The state of California will consider a statewide version of the San Francisco ban in the 2007 legislative session.

Steps you can take to reduce exposure to phthalates:

- Avoid vinyl shower curtains and other products made of PVC plastic (#3).

- Stop giving children soft vinyl toys made with phthalates. Look for products labeled "PVC free", "Fragrance free" or products without that "shower curtain smell."

- Don't microwave food for your child in plastic containers; use glass.

- Limit your use of phthalate-containing personal care products, especially for small children or if you are pregnant. Avoid products with the word "fragrance" on the label.

- A quick Internet search will bring up sites describing products you can purchase that are free of these chemicals.

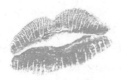

# 3

## *Because We're Worth It!*

Janet Nudelman was the right person to call on the world's largest cosmetics companies to stop using chemicals suspected of causing cancer and birth defects. As program director of the Breast Cancer Fund, she had the resources and a bit of moral authority to back her up. Plus, unlike many environmentalists in the nonprofit sector, Janet had a background in corporate America. She'd spent four years as political director of the phone company Working Assets.

"I already knew that it was possible for companies to be sustainable and do the right thing. I knew that companies weren't all necessarily black and white, that there were a lot of shades of gray within the corporate community," Janet said. "So I went out with this naïve kind of attitude, which was like, well, why *wouldn't* you want to do the right thing? Why wouldn't you want to take toxic chemicals out of cosmetics if there were safer alternatives available, particularly if women's health was at risk? And I think that really served me, because I was pretty fearless when it came to talking with the big companies."

The timing was right, too. The third largest environmental group in the US, Friends of the Earth (FOE), had just completed a five-year strategic plan and decided to prioritize work on cancer prevention. They wanted to partner with the Breast Cancer Fund to bring together major environmental and health groups to create the first-ever national cancer prevention project. About 40 groups attended the first meeting of the National Alliance for Cancer Prevention in Washington DC in the spring of 2003. There was a lot of interest in collaborating, but the groups needed a concrete project to work on. "We realized pretty quickly that it's hard to organize people around a concept," Janet recalled.

Charlotte Brody and Bryony Schwan had just the concrete project: cosmetics. Their *Not Too Pretty* report had generated hundreds of media stories and thousands of e-mails from women who were concerned about toxic chemicals in cosmetics and who wanted the FDA to take action. But they needed more groups to get involved in order to create sustained political pressure. So they pitched the idea to the executive committee of the National Alliance for Cancer Prevention. "About half of the people immediately said yes, this seems like a great opportunity," Janet Nudelman said, "and the other half said no, we don't want to put our energies there." Some groups thought cosmetics were "too frivolous

## Andrea's Story

Some people take the mean embers of adversity and transmute them into a wildfire for change. That was Andrea Martin, who founded the Breast Cancer Fund in her living room after getting her second breast cancer diagnosis.

At age 42, Andrea was diagnosed with stage-three breast cancer that had spread to her lymph nodes. She was told she had little chance of survival and advised to put her affairs in order. But after a year of grueling treatment, Andrea was in recovery. She took a job as deputy finance director for Diane Feinstein's 1992 campaign for the US Senate. Two months into the campaign, Andrea found the lump in her remaining breast. The first cancer caused her to feel afraid; the second cancer sparked the outrage that created the Breast Cancer Fund. From her living room, Andrea wrote letters to everyone she knew — college friends, former colleagues, doctors, fellow cancer survivors, political connections — asking for money to fund research and patient support programs for breast cancer. She was also intent on raising the question of cause: why were so many women getting breast cancer? Andrea spearheaded the first international science summit and commissioned the first scientific report on the environmental causes of breast cancer.

Under her leadership, the Breast Cancer Fund grew into a national advocacy force with more than 70,000 supporters and a reputation for cutting-edge ☞

of an issue" to work on, or that the science wasn't strong enough because not much was known at the time about which chemicals were in cosmetics.

From a breast cancer perspective, the idea was intriguing. New research was showing that exposure to hormone-disrupting chemicals, especially during sensitive times of breast development such as in the womb and during puberty, could increase the risk of breast cancer. Teenagers and pregnant women were two groups likely to be exposed to hormonally active ingredients in cosmetics. Janet also saw cosmetics as a tangible and personal way to tell the story about chemical exposure. "It was clear to me that we could use the whole notion of safe cosmetics as a vehicle to talk about cancer prevention and the need to take a precautionary approach toward chemicals," she said.

The Breast Cancer Fund, along with several other groups in the Alliance — Friends of the Earth, the National Black Environmental Justice Coalition, National Environmental Trust and Alliance for Healthy

research into less-toxic treatments, alternatives to mammography and prevention of the disease. After almost ten years at the helm of the Breast Cancer Fund, Andrea had another fateful trip to the doctor's office and another horrible diagnosis. She learned she had a malignant brain tumor, which the doctors suspected was caused by radiation treatments for the breast cancer. She had emergency brain surgery, but the prognosis was grim.

In one of her last activist projects, Andrea's photo appeared in a full-age ad in the *New York Times* and she flew to Washington, DC to speak at a press conference organized by the Environmental Working Group. She had been among the Commonweal Cohort, the first nine people in the world to know their personal chemical body burden from their participation in the EWG/Mount Sinai study.[1] "Warning, Andrea Martin contains 59 cancer causing chemicals," read the headline over her photo in the ad.[2] "My body biology is susceptible to cancer," Andrea said. Did she think her chemical body burden contributed to the cancer? "No one can say for sure. But no one can say it hasn't," she said. "We deserve to know what toxins are in our bodies. We have a right to know what health effects these chemicals have."[3] Andrea died shortly afterward at the age of 57, but her fire burns on in what is today the only national organization focused solely on preventing breast cancer by identifying and eliminating the environmental causes of the disease.

Tomorrow — decided to join forces with the authors of the *Not Too Pretty* report to create a national cosmetics campaign. The founding groups met at the FOE offices in February 2004 and decided to call their new project "Because We're Worth It! The Campaign for Safe Cosmetics." The words of the new logo were underlined in lipstick red. They printed up T-shirts, designed their first brochure and rushed to put together a website in time for their first public outing.

## Be Safe, Healthy and Free!

April 25, 2004 — The crowd stood shoulder to shoulder from the Lincoln Memorial to the steps of the US Capitol in what organizers called the largest march on Washington in history. More than one million people joined the March for Women's Lives, the first rally focused on women's reproductive freedom since 1992. Significantly and largely due to the organizing efforts of African-American and Latina women, the march focused not just on abortion rights, but on the broader theme of women's health, including access to health care, contraception, sex education and global family planning.

Lisa Archer, the new grassroots organizer for the Campaign for Safe Cosmetics, thought the women's march was the perfect place to debut the campaign's message of toxic-free products and toxic-free bodies. The work was closer to her heart than most people knew. Though raised in rural Wyoming, Lisa had long worried about the environmental problems of the world. The issues really hit home when, at age 12, she learned her mother had breast cancer. "How could this be happening?" Lisa wondered. "There's no breast cancer in the family. I realized, more and more families are dealing with this — with mothers, sisters, grandmothers and daughters being struck with this disease. It's a true epidemic." In college, Lisa delved into environmental health studies, women's studies and social justice issues, learning all she could. "I realized it's all connected. We look at these issues as though they are separate, but they're all connected," Lisa said.

That day at the March for Women's Lives, behind the ten-foot-long banner emblazoned with the words "Because We're Worth It!" Lisa was marching for everything she cared about, alongside a million other advocates for women's rights. Removing toxic chemicals from personal care products is "a battle of fertility too," she explained. "It's all about, will we have healthy families? Will we be able to have healthy daughters and sons when we choose to? This is fundamentally about our ability to have healthy and fulfilling lives."

## Company Roll Call

The Campaign for Safe Cosmetics' first goal, to get cosmetics companies to stop using chemicals linked to cancer and birth defects, fit right in with Lisa's vision. But it wasn't going to be easy. A year earlier, Bryony Schwan had placed more than 30 phone calls from her office in Missoula, Montana, to the five top cosmetics companies. She wanted to know: since the companies had to reformulate their European products to remove the two phthalates DEHP and DBP, would they please make the phthalate-free products available in the US?

To sum up the companies' responses: "They blew me off, totally." Bryony's notes record: seven calls to Unilever, six calls to L'Oréal, eight calls to Revlon, seven calls to Estée Lauder. The only phone responses were from L'Oréal vice president of communications Sam Maddingly and Revlon spokeswoman Catherine Fisher, both of whom said they'd call back but never did. Estée Lauder sent a form letter written by the trade association saying phthalates are safe. After four phone calls to Procter & Gamble, Bryony managed to get a phone meeting with company executives. During the call, P&G spokesperson and toxicologist Dr. Tim Long explained the company's position that phthalates are safe. He told Bryony at one point that American women aren't as concerned about cosmetics safety as the Europeans.[4]

Janet Nudelman was getting ready to convince the companies otherwise — this time with a letter signed by 60 women's and environmental groups under the letterhead of the Breast Cancer Fund. The letter explained the European Union's new Cosmetics Directive and asked the companies to sign a Compact for Safe Cosmetics, a pledge to replace hazardous chemicals with safer alternatives within three years.

The Compact for Safe Cosmetics asked companies to do four things:

1. Remove EU-banned chemicals from all products sold anywhere in the world.
2. Inventory all products for chemicals of concern, including ingredients that are persistent, bio-accumulative, toxic to the brain or reproductive system, carcinogenic, mutagenic, endocrine disrupters or sensitizers.

3. Develop a plan to substitute hazardous chemicals with safer alternatives within three years.
4. Publicly report on progress.

Janet mailed the letters off to 250 companies in February of 2004 and eagerly awaited the responses. The first, dated March 30, was short and to the point. "The Estée Lauder Companies Inc. and its brands fully support the position and statement attached from the Cosmetic, Toiletry, and Fragrance Association. Thank you for your understanding in this matter."[5] The attached statement from the CTFA said the European Union's new Cosmetics Directive (which banned 1,100 ingredients from cosmetics) "represents an unnecessary change in the philosophy of regulations of cosmetic ingredients in the EU. First of all, it may remove valuable ingredients from use in the EU. In addition, it ignores exposure information that would be used to assess whether there could be any harm from the use of such ingredients." The statement explained that in the US the cosmetics industry and FDA work together to ensure the safety of products. "The bottom line for American consumers is that they are just as protected as consumers in Europe and have products that are just as safe."[6]

Janet was disappointed, even surprised. She had harbored hopes that Estée Lauder — whose "pink ribbon" public relations campaigns raise money for breast cancer research — would step up to the plate as an industry leader. But it didn't happen. Revlon was next to send the CTFA statement: phthalates are safe and the EU regulations unnecessary. In April and May, more letters started coming in the door. Janet kept meticulous track of the responses in a spread sheet. Gap Inc. would globally reformulate their products to remove chemicals banned in Europe but couldn't sign the Compact because they "rely on government agencies to determine the safety of approved ingredients in a scientific and consistent manner."[7] Coty Inc. would also globally reformulate but "cannot assume third party timelines and substitution plans" as requested by the Compact.[8] Custom Esthetics Ltd. already didn't use EU-banned chemicals, but "corporate policy discourages us from joining advocacy groups that solicit our alliance."[9] Blistex Inc. respectfully declined to either reformulate globally or sign the Compact.[10]

Some positive responses started trickling in as well. Osea, an all-natural skin care company, was the first to sign the Compact for Safe Cosmetics, followed by a handful of others. The tone of these letters was distinctly different, friendly and even welcoming. Within a few months, 35 companies had signed the Compact for Safe Cosmetics, all of them smaller companies from the natural products industry.

## Eternity Moment

The campaign had made special efforts to get the attention of mega-corporation Unilever. Besides Bryony's seven phone calls and Janet's letter, there was a quarter-page ad that ran in the *Washington Post* the day the Cosmetic Ingredient Review panel made its decision about phthalates. "Something has come between me and my Calvins," said the ad, urging the FDA and companies to take action to remove phthalates from personal care products. "Calvin Klein's Eternity. Aqua Net Hair Spray. Salon Selectives Hair Mousse. Dove Solid Anti-Perspirant. All these cosmetics and beauty aids have two things in common. They're manufactured by Unilever, the Dutch-based consumer products conglomerate. And they all contain toxic chemicals called phthalates (THA-lates)."[11]

Unilever had yet to reply to the campaign. When a campaign volunteer named Mary Anne Dixon e-mailed Unilever to ask if she was better off buying the European version of her favorite Dove body wash, she got this response:

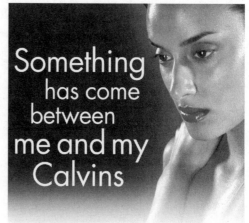

**Something has come between me and my Calvins**

**Toxic chemicals in beauty care products.**

Calvin Klein's Eternity. Aqua Net Hair Spray. Salon Selectives Hair Mousse. Dove Solid Anti-Perspirant.

All these cosmetics and beauty aids have two things in common.

They're manufactured by Unilever, the Dutch-based consumer products conglomerate.

And they all contain toxic chemicals called phthalates (THA-lates).

Phthalates have been shown to damage the lung, liver and kidneys, and to harm the developing testes of male offspring.

These results come from animal tests which, according to government scientists, are relevant to predicting health impacts in humans.

Last week, the European Union ordered a phase-out of two phthalates in cosmetic and beauty products.

Today, the U.S. Cosmetics Ingredient Review Panel will decide whether American consumers will be protected.

Safe alternatives to phthalates are already being used in many beauty products. Now is the time for the federal government—and for companies like Calvin Klein and Unilever—to act decisively.

After all, Eternity is a long time.

**Learn more at www.NotTooPretty.org**

This ad sponsored by Women's Voices for the Earth, Environmental Working Group and Health Care Without Harm

Women's Voices for the Earth, 114 West Pine Street, Missoula, MT 59802

FENTON

*This ad ran in the* Washington Post *on the same day the industry's self-policing Cosmetic Ingredient Review panel ruled that phthalates are "safe as currently used."*

*Hi Mary Anne,*

*Thanks for writing! We have no information on this subject. Products from other countries may have some different ingredients because of what is best for their environment. United States has the safest products that our laws will allow both for the consumer and the environment. Please be assured, we would not allow a product to be sold if there was any danger in harming anyone.*

*Thank you for your interest!*
*Your friends at Unilever Bestfoods* [12]

When Karen Stanston wrote to ask about Eternity perfume, Marie Stuart of Consumer Affairs wrote back: "We are aware of the public concerns about the safety of phthalates and take them very seriously. We use only those phthalates that are important components of our products and have been shown to be safe by scientific risk assessment." [13] Stuart explained that the major phthalate used in Unilever products is diethyl phthalate (DEP), used in low levels as a "bittering agent" to make alcohol undrinkable in products such as aftershaves, in accordance with FDA regulations. She recommended visiting the industry trade association website for more information about phthalates.

"We do hope this information will allow you to continue enjoying the classic and timeless scent of ETERNITY without further concern," Stuart wrote. "In addition, we would be delighted to share with you a complimentary sample of Calvin Klein's newest fragrance: the playful, sophisticated and ultra-feminine ETERNITY MOMENT. A scent that captures the excitement and exhilaration of falling in love. A modern, fresh-squeezed floral, the multi-textured fragrance bursts with succulent beauty in notes like Pomegranate Flower, Chinese Pink Peony, Passion Flower and Raspberry Cashmere ... Just one MOMENT can change everything!"

In South Korea, Unilever was responding quite differently to consumer concerns. The Women's Committee of the Korean Federation for Environmental Movements had decided to do their own product testing to look for phthalates in cosmetics. They bought 24 products in various famous department stores throughout Seoul and sent them to a lab. "All of the products investigated had phthalates. Hundred percent of the products investigated, i.e. perfume, hair mousse, hair spray, hair coloring and nail polish, contained phthalates," said the group's April 2003 report. "Ninety-six percent of the investigated products contained more than two kinds of phthalates, 50% had more than three kinds, and 8% had four different kinds." [14]

The Women's Committee marched down to Unilever Korea headquarters and demanded the removal of phthalates. The company responded in writing: "Our firm does not use DEHP and DBP, about which concerns have been raised, as components of our products," said the letter from Tae-Hyun Chang, director of the Central Research Center of Unilever Korea.[15] Although the company had been using the phthalate DEP as a component in fragrance, they had found a way to remove even that chemical, Chang said. They would gradually introduce the new formula starting at the end of the year.

According to Chang, Unilever Korea had also begun testing containers to make sure phthalates were not leaching from the plastic, and they were working with the cosmetics industry trade association in Korea to prepare voluntary agreements about phthalates. "Through continuous improvement of product quality in our firm, we will do our best to develop products that consumers can use safely. Our company will become even more reliable," Chang wrote. In just a few months, the Women's Committee had scored a major victory for safer products in South Korea. But more than a year after the release of the *Not Too Pretty* report, the US environmental groups still couldn't get a response from the Dutch conglomerate.

## Power of the Press

Procter & Gamble — creator of such iconic symbols to American womanhood as Tide, Crest, Ivory and Cover Girl — was also singing a different tune to consumers overseas. The company's official position, as P&G spokesperson Tim Long told Bryony Schwan, was that phthalates are safe as currently used in cosmetics. But a conflicting message appeared to be coming out of the company's UK office. The letter was on Procter & Gamble UK letterhead from the office in Newcastle upon Tyne. It was addressed to Helen Lynn of the Women's Environmental Network

(WEN), a co-author of the European *Pretty Nasty* report. "We agree with WEN's position on the inherent toxicological potential of Di (2 ethylhexyl) phthalate (DEHP) and Dibutyl phthalate (DBP)," wrote Kathy Rogerson, P&G technical external relations. "We take a precautionary approach and will only use an ingredient if it is safe and approved for use in Cosmetic products. As a consequence of this approach, there is already a program to remove DEHP and DBP from our products." [16]

A reporter from the *Wall Street Journal* was interested in the letter from Kathy Rogerson — and just like that, there was big news in the $650 million American nail-care market: "Amid Health Concerns, Nail-Polish Makers Switch Formulas," read the headline of the April 19, 2004, story by Thaddeus Herrick. [17] "At least two major cosmetics makers are phasing out use of a common chemical in nail polish that has emerged as a health concern, especially for women in their childbearing years," Herrick wrote. "Procter & Gamble Co. said it will reformulate its Max Factor and Cover Girl polishes and Estée Lauder Cos. said it will redo its Clinique and MAC lines, among others, to eliminate the chemical in the US."

Both companies had already removed the chemical in Europe, the article explained, due to Europe's precautionary approach toward chemicals. "While US regulators tend to wait for clear evidence of problems, the EU has been moving aggressively to remove chemicals with the potential for trouble," Herrick wrote. But both companies were careful to say their decision to remove DBP had nothing to do with health concerns. P&G spokesman Tim Long said they would remove DBP "because consumers prefer the performance of the alternative already introduced in Europe." Estée Lauder spokeswoman Janet Bartucci said their decision was due to a company policy to use the same ingredients worldwide. Unilever — confronted by Herrick with their contradictory letter from South Korea — said it was not planning to reformulate products in the US to remove DBP. In a written response to the newspaper, "Unilever North America said it believes phthalates are safe, as does the Cosmetic Ingredient Review panel. Unilever didn't address the Korea memo," Herrick wrote.

## Who Owns Your Worth?

Sometimes the truth is even more surreal than the glossy ads. That's what it felt like the day the letter arrived from L'Oréal. The French cosmetics titan had not responded to the Breast Cancer Fund letter, but they had something else to say to the Campaign for Safe Cosmetics. The message was from the Paul Hastings, Janofsky & Walker LLP firm in New York.

*Dear Madame: We represent L'Oréal and write to you in connection with the Safe Cosmetics Action Network. It recently was brought to our attention that your organization uses the slogan BECAUSE WE'RE WORTH IT! on its website and to identify its Campaign for Safe Cosmetics. As you no doubt are aware, for nearly thirty years, L'Oréal's signature slogan has been BECAUSE YOU'RE WORTH IT. L'Oréal owns federal trademark registrations not only for BECAUSE YOU'RE WORTH IT, but also for BECAUSE I'M WORTH IT and BECAUSE WE'RE WORTH IT, TOO! Your organization's use of BECAUSE WE'RE WORTH IT cannot help but cause confusion as to source, sponsorship, endorsement or affiliation with L'Oréal.*[18]

The letter "should not be interpreted as complaining about the campaign itself or your website," Sherman wrote, "it merely requires you to remove the slogan BECAUSE WE'RE WORTH IT!" from all materials within ten days in order to avoid further consequences.

What to do now was a point of heated debate within the Campaign for Safe Cosmetics. The slogan was not exactly L'Oréal's trademark, but a slight variation of it — *we're* worth it, instead of *you're* worth it, or *I'm* worth it. Did that make a difference? The lawyers at the Breast Cancer Fund didn't think so. Still, it felt funny not to be allowed to use those four little words in public. Could it really be illegal to declare self-worth? Some of us wanted to fight for the slogan. In the end, the lawyers advised the Breast Cancer Fund, the campaign's fiscal sponsor, not to pit their $3-million-a-year budget against the world's largest cosmetics company. So off came the slogan from the logo, the website and the materials. The T-shirts created for the March for Women's Lives became contraband; the lawyers warned us never to wear them in public.

And off went a new letter to L'Oréal: "Prior to adopting the campaign name *Because We're Worth It! The Campaign for Safe Cosmetics,* we conducted a thorough internet search and found hundreds of uses of that slogan in diverse sources, including British Broadcasting Corp., a television series exploring globalization, a children's book on self esteem, a Star Wars website, a British firefighters' union and a Nurse & Midwives fair pay campaign." Nevertheless, the campaign removed the slogan at L'Oréal's request and now had a few requests for L'Oréal in return. The letter requested a meeting with company officials to discuss nine L'Oréal products — three that contained the EU-banned phthalates and six that contained known or probable carcinogens according to a new report by the Environmental Working Group. "We trust that, as the world's largest manufacturer of cosmetics, L'Oréal too would like to see a world in which the entire cosmetics industry produces cosmetics and personal care products free from known or suspected carcinogens, mutagens or reproductive toxins," concluded the letter.[19] L'Oréal representatives wrote to explain that their products were already safe and in compliance with the intent of the campaign's request. It was going to take more than a letter to get the French titan's attention.

## No More Shades of Gray

Janet Nudelman was starting to see a different side of corporate America than she'd experienced over at Working Assets. "I was just shocked when they would bold faced turn around and say 'No, we're not going to do this. We believe our definitions of safe are safe enough and we don't care if there's conflicting scientific evidence,'" Janet said. "They weren't engaging in a real dialogue with us, and that was their loss. That was a really big loss as far as I'm concerned, because we weren't trying to nail them to the cross. We really approached these companies I think in good faith, and asked them to be leaders within their industries on behalf of the issue. But pretty quickly the big companies started peeling away, you know, walking away from the light to the dark side." Janet still shakes her head at L'Oréal's demand to stop using the "Because We're Worth It!" slogan. "The really ironic thing about that is, if anything, it would reflect well on them, not badly, because people would see the relationship between safe cosmetics and L'Oréal, not the opposite."

As the major multinationals distanced themselves from the Campaign for Safe Cosmetics and stood behind the Cosmetic, Toiletry, and Fragrance Association, the smaller companies were sidling up. "The numbers almost ran parallel," Janet said. "As the number of conventional companies that refused to have anything to do with this issue or the campaign increased, the number of natural products companies that wanted to align themselves with the goals and values of the campaign increased simultaneously." A year after her initial letter went out, 70 companies had signed the Compact for Safe Cosmetics.

Within six months, the number doubled, and in another six months, it doubled again. By early 2007, more than 500 companies — including more than 90 outside the US — had signed the safe cosmetics pledge.

Notably, all the signers were natural products companies. Not one major conventional company was on the list.

## Undercover, Part I

Which cosmetics company do you trust with your daughter? The campaign decided to put the question to the public in a full-page ad in *USA Today*. "Putting on Makeup Shouldn't be like Playing with Matches," said the headline over the photo of the little girl smearing lipstick on her face.[20] The ad named three companies that had not yet publicly committed to remove the EU-banned ingredients globally — Unilever, Revlon and L'Oréal. "Ask them to join the growing number of toxin-free cosmetics companies and regain the trust of American women," said the ad, which ran on the same day the cosmetics industry was gathering in Manhattan for its largest conference of the year.

Susan Roll, an organizer with the Campaign for Safe Cosmetics, brought several copies of *USA Today* with her to the Health and Beauty America 2004 conference. The 35-year-old breast cancer activist had never infiltrated an industry conference before, and she was worried that someone might see through her fake business cards that said she was a beauty consultant for a fictitious company named Joyful. But she was also excited. She was finally going to get a close-up look at the industry she'd been tracking for a year in her job as associate executive director of the Massachusetts Breast Cancer Coalition.

When no one was looking, Susan dropped a copy of *USA Today* here and there — on the table near the entrance, on the bench in the ladies' room — opened to the page with the photo of the little girl smearing on lipstick. In one bathroom, she met a woman who was so thrilled with the name of Susan's pretend company, Joyful, that she wanted to use it as an example during a marketing session she was giving later that day. "Sure," Susan said smiling, explaining that Joy is her middle name. She took one last look in the mirror to check her makeup — she wasn't used to wearing so much of it — and headed off to the panel called "US and International Issues Affecting Cosmetics and OTC Drugs" organized by the Cosmetic, Toiletry, and Fragrance Association.

The "issues affecting cosmetics" were of a regulatory nature, and the new European Union Cosmetics Directive was causing quite a buzz in a room. Susan sat in the back and tried to look inconspicuous. When CTFA president Ed Kavanaugh asked how many companies would be affected by the new European regulations, three quarters of the people raised their hands. "We are the most unregulated industry under the auspices of the FDA and this makes us vulnerable," Kavanaugh said.[21] It was clear that the role of CTFA was to keep it that way. Thomas Donegan, vice president of legal and general counsel at CTFA, explained how the US regulatory system works for cosmetics. Donegan

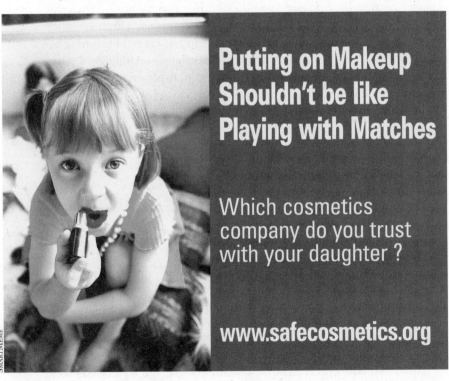

*This image was displayed at the Cannes Film Festival in France. A version also ran in*
USA Today.

described cosmetics as "an easy entry business" with no pre-market approval necessary.

When asked by an audience member how FDA determines if a cosmetic product is "safe," Donegan explained: "This is left to the company. If a company says their product is safe, it can go on the market." But things were changing in Europe with the Seventh Amendment to the Cosmetics Directive, as Andreas Mestel from the European trade association explained. He said companies were not likely to be given a grace period in removing the banned ingredients, since everyone had known about the new regulations for two years. Susan wrote in her notes, "Mestel feels as though regulations are getting stricter worldwide and will continue to do so. CTFA made it clear that they will continue to fight stricter regulations."

Next up was Gerald McEwan, CTFA vice president of science, and the topic turned to the other pest buzzing in the room that day, the Campaign for Safe Cosmetics. Susan had a hard time staying in her seat. McEwan, she said later, was "very derogatory, almost making fun of us like we were little kids out of our league, and who did we think we were taking them on." But she stayed put, scribbling notes furiously. McEwan said that phthalates are being used by advocates to attack the industry, and he identified Health Care Without Harm as one of the "biggest problems" on the use of phthalates. Advocates were now using the EU Cosmetics Directive to force industry's hand, McEwan said. He reminded everyone that the US Cosmetic Ingredient Review panel concluded phthalates are safe.

"They just want all plastic out," McEwan said of the advocates. "They twist the statements of our companies. They are still after us." California, in particular, was a problem. McEwan reported that two bills on cosmetics safety had been defeated, and he was especially proud of the industry's response to Assemblywoman Wilma Chan's bill that would have banned DEHP and DBP from cosmetics sold in California. He explained that CTFA had someone testify with a basket of fruits, vegetables and a bottle of water, and suggest how ridiculous it would be to test everything that goes into our bodies. It was an effective and compelling argument, he said. "Our adversaries were upset and surprised," McEwan said, but he warned they would be back with more attempts to increase regulations. The adversaries are "strong, competent, smart and well-financed" — as evidenced by the ad in *USA Today.* "It is all on their website, safecosmetics.org. It is a very impressive website and it tells everything that they are working on. I encourage all of you to visit it. Be sure your name is not listed."

## A Little Bit Safer

After *USA Today* hit the stands with the full-page ad of the little girl smearing on lipstick, it took all of about two hours for Revlon communication director Catherine Fisher to contact the Campaign for Safe Cosmetics — the same Catherine Fisher who promised Bryony Schwan 18 months earlier that she'd call back, but never did. Fisher complained that the ad misrepresented Revlon because the company's products already did meet the EU standards worldwide. Janet Nudelman asked for confirmation in writing.

Within two months, Revlon, L'Oréal and Unilever sent written confirmation that their products would be reformulated worldwide to remove the EU-banned chemicals. A handful of hazardous ingredients were on their way out of products made by several of the world's largest cosmetics companies. The Campaign for Safe Cosmetics raised a torch of victory. But the games were just beginning.

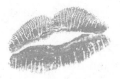

# 4

# Skin Deeper

So what else is in cosmetics? Jane Houlihan wanted to know. She knew it wasn't going to be an easy question to answer. There was no central list of all the chemicals used in personal care products, for one thing, and no systematic way to check ingredients for health concerns. The information lived in bits and pieces all over the place. What if she could pull it all together and make it easily accessible to the public?

Some ideas strike like lightning, but this one started rising slowly like the sun during a plane journey to California. Jane Houlihan had just settled in for the cross-country flight and cracked open the not-so-light reading she'd brought along for the ride: a two-inch-thick softcover called the *Cosmetic Ingredient Review Compendium*.[1] The book, which she'd ordered online for $350 plus $10 shipping and handling, contained safety summaries of 1,100 ingredients reviewed by the cosmetic industry's safety panel in its 30-year history. "I just started reading it, and as I'm going through, reading summary after summary, I'm barely through the As and into the Bs and Cs, when I realize that this summary is just a gold mine of information on the safety of chemicals that are specifically in cosmetics. It exists nowhere else," Jane said.

She noticed one thing right away: for a lot of the chemicals the safety panel had reviewed, their conclusion was that they didn't have enough data to know if an ingredient was safe. For some chemicals, the panel had decided ingredients were unsafe and shouldn't be used in certain applications. "So as I was reading through, I quickly grabbed onto the idea that we could turn this into a database, compare it back to ingredients in products and see if the industry is even following the recommendations of their own safety manual," Jane said. She pulled out her laptop and started typing data into a spreadsheet.

## If She Builds It

Back at the Washington DC offices of the Environmental Working Group, where a banner with the slogan "The Power of Information" hangs in the entranceway, Jane kept working on the spreadsheet, her idea rising higher. "Once I realized that maybe we did have a systematic way to evaluate ingredient safety, we needed to build up a database of ingredients in products," she explained. Nobody in the entire multi-billion-dollar cosmetics industry had a comprehensive list of ingredients in cosmetic products — or if they did they weren't sharing it.

Jane put staffers to work searching for ingredient lists. They pulled product ingredients from websites like drugstore.com and alta.com which specialize in online cosmetics sales. For some brands not sold online (such as Estée Lauder and Avon), they bought products and entered ingredients by hand or contacted the companies. As an example of how difficult it could be to get information: volunteers with Women's Voices for the Earth spent months e-mailing Estée Lauder to ask for product ingredients — for two products at a time, since that's all the company would release in a single e-mail. It was tedious work. And the product ingredients were only half the challenge.

For the other half of what was to become a report called *Skin Deep*, EWG needed to pull together as many credible sources of information as they could find about the toxicity and health impacts of chemicals. They tracked down lists of known and suspected chemical health hazards from various government and academic sources — lists from the US FDA, EPA, National Toxicology Program, European Chemical Bureau and peer-reviewed academic journals — and merged them together into a common database.

If you'd expect the cosmetics industry to have a central list of product ingredients, you might suppose the government would already have a central database of hazard information about chemicals. But Jane's new tool — 15 toxicity databases merged together, later expanded to 37 and then 50 — was the only one of its kind in the world. It wasn't the first time EWG had done the government's job. The nonprofit group also built the Farm Subsidy Database[2] that tracks billions of dollars paid in government farm subsidies so anyone can go online and find out who gets the checks. EWG liked to tell the story about the time the US Department of Agriculture called them to ask for a sort on the database.

*The Power of Information.* The goal of the Environmental Working Group is to shine light on industry and government dealings and empower the public with facts. When complete, *Skin Deep* would score thousands of personal care products for toxicity and show safer alternatives in each product category. It would be the only tool of its kind. But first, a lot of not-so-glamorous work had to happen. The science databases, which spoke various languages of government and academic sources, needed to be able to talk to each other. "They talk by understanding the ingredients, by having consistent ingredient names," Jane explained. "That step was extraordinarily laborious because there are so many different ways to denote or spell the same chemical." Witch hazel, for instance, had at least seven different spellings of its two botanical names, used in various combinations. Each variation had to be fixed by hand so the names were consistent — for thousands of ingredients. "We'd lose interns over it, and then we'd bring in new interns," Jane said. They got good at figuring out which interns would have the stamina to stay the longest.

The initial team at EWG included former meteorologist and database architect Sean Gray, toxicologist Dr. Tim Kropp and two Web designers. Product by product, they marked down package directions for intended use and checked toxicity scores for errors "until you practically go blind," explained Hema Subramanian, who worked on the database for two years after the initial launch. "There is a strict protocol for categorizing the products and maintaining quality control. It's a grueling task and repetitive, but it's important for someone to do the legwork. You can't just automate it, there's no way."

Finally, in the spring of 2004, the day came when the databases were finished and it was time to merge the two halves of *Skin Deep*[3] — thousands of products matched up against more than a dozen databases of chemical hazards. "This was like the wedding," Jane recalled with a shine in her eyes. "You marry the product ingredient database to all toxicity databases and see where they match up. It was exciting. It was just an extraordinary list of findings."

## Message in a Bottle

The first thing Jane Houlihan noticed was that some brands were using ingredients in ways the industry's own safety panel said were unsafe, or were using ingredients for which they didn't have enough data to know if the uses were safe. "That to me was the biggest irony: that this industry that is purportedly self regulating, that pushed 30 years ago to have their own safety panel outside of FDA, was not even following the advice of that panel when it comes to product safety," Jane said.

For example, Destin Diaper Rash Ointment, Creamy, Fresh Scent contained sodium borate, an ingredient that "should not be used on infant skin or injured skin." Klear Action Acne Treatment System contained ceteareth-20, an ingredient that "should not be used on damaged skin." Pond's Clear Solutions Overnight Blemish Reducers contained butyl methacrylate, which "should be accompanied with directions to avoid skin contact."[4] Besides such renegade products, "it was fascinating to see where the toxicities aligned," Jane said. "Personal care products contain carcinogens, pesticides, reproductive toxins, endocrine disruptors, plasticizers, degreasers and surfactants." The chemical industry in a bottle, she called it.

*Skin Deep*'s findings in 2005 included:

- ⅓ of personal care products contain at least one ingredient linked to cancer.
- 45% of products contain an ingredient that may be harmful to the reproductive system or to a baby's development.
- 60% of products contain chemicals that can act like estrogen or disrupt hormones in the body.
- 56% of products contain "penetration enhancer" chemicals, which help other chemicals penetrate faster and deeper into the body.
- 87% of ingredients in personal care products have not been assessed for safety by the Cosmetic Ingredient Review, the industry's self-policing safety panel.[5]

## Not So Pure and Clean

*Pure, clean, gentle.* There's hardly a product label that doesn't use these words. Yet according to *Skin Deep*, up to 80% of products may contain one or more hidden hazards that are not even listed on product labels. Recent product tests chronicled in the book *Safe Trip to Eden* by David Steinman shed light on this problem with cosmetics safety.[6]

Busy with three kids, David Steinman's wife didn't have time to worry about toxic products. So he worried for them all. "Maybe it's because I know too many secrets," he said. For instance, the leading baby product line is Johnson & Johnson's, whose website says its products are clinically tested to ensure they are "mild and gentle enough for newborns." As David explained in his book, this is why the company replaced the harsh cleanser sodium *lauryl* sulfate with the much gentler sodium *laureth* sulfate.[7] Lauryl is converted to laureth by adding the petrochemical ethylene oxide. But this process — called ethoxylation — creates the petroleum-derived contaminant 1,4-dioxane, a known animal and probable human carcinogen according to the EPA.

In 2002, David Steinman started buying personal care products that contain ethoxylated ingredients and sending them to a lab to test for 1,4-dioxane. The lab found the cancer-causing chemical in 18 of two dozen products tested, including 15 popular baby shampoos and bath products.[8] The contaminant was not listed on any of the labels.

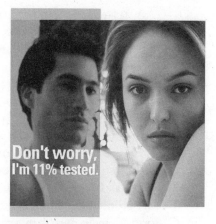

*A version of this ad ran in* USA Today, *pointing out that only 11% of cosmetic ingredients have been reviewed by the industry safety panel, based on the 2005* Skin Deep *report.*

The manufacturers claim the levels are too low to cause harm. However, low levels of exposure can add up. The same infant exposed to 1,4-dioxane from the Grins and Giggles baby shampoo could also be exposed to the carcinogen from the Tigger bath bubbles and the Clean as Can Bee body wash in a single bath — as well as from food, water and other household products in the same day. "It's these multiple exposures to carcinogens that are cause for concern, especially for developing children," said Janet Nudelman from the Breast Cancer Fund. "We have to ask, is it necessary for baby shampoos to contain cancer-causing chemicals at all? The answer is no." For minimal cost, 1,4-dioxane can be vacuum stripped out of products at the end of the manufacturing process to non-detectable levels — or avoided entirely by using ingredients that do not need to be ethoxylated. But the companies are not required to do so. According to an analysis of *Skin Deep*, 97% of hair straighteners, 57% of baby soaps and 36% of facial creams contain petrochemical ingredients that may be contaminated with 1,4-dioxane.[9]

Unfortunately, when it comes to carcinogenic contaminants in personal care products, 1,4-dioxane is just the tip of the iceberg. An EWG analysis shows that one of every five adults is potentially exposed every day to all of the top seven carcinogenic impurities common to personal care product ingredients — hydroquinone, ethylene oxide, 1,4-dioxane, formaldehyde, nitrosamines, PAHs and acrylamide.[10]

## For Sensitive Skin

Laura Jones doesn't want to think about how much cash she plunked down at the Sephora store in Washington DC's swanky Georgetown neighborhood. Eye glitter, lip gloss, high-end perfume — she kept her investments in a huge silver toolbox that her friends envied. They often asked her for makeup advice, since Laura knew just about everything there was to know about application techniques and product performance. What she didn't know was that she was allergic to most of her favorite products. In her mid 20s, Laura began noticing that her face turned red and developed bumps after exercising or drinking wine. "Basically anytime I got flushed, I looked like a beet," she recalled.

Her primary care physician prescribed a skin cream that Laura later discovered was a topical steroid. While the drug initially improved the sensitivity, the redness problem kept getting worse. She kept using more skin products to try to cover up the problem — cleansers, toners, scrubs and defoliators along with her usual four hair products and full-face makeup. "It became a vicious cycle where my skin was ruddy and uneven looking and so I used more makeup to cover up the irritation that the products were causing."

Eventually, Laura found a dermatologist who weaned her off the face steroids and conducted patch tests that found she was allergic to common ingredients in her products, including fragrance and formaldehyde-releaser preservatives. Laura embarked on a quest to find products she could use. ☛

## Hold the Carcinogens Please

Since they are not listed on labels, there is no way to know which personal care products contain impurities. But many ingredients may be contaminated.

- 1,4-dioxane may be present in detergents and shampoos that contain the following ingredients or partial ingredient names: sodium laureth sulfate, PEG, polyethylene, polyethylene glycol, polyoxyethylene, polysorbate, -eth- or -oxynol-.

- The following ingredients contain formaldehyde, may release formaldehyde or may break down into formaldehyde: 2-bromo-2-nitropropane-1,3-diol; diazolidinyl urea; DMDM hydantoin; imidazolidinyl urea; quaternium-15.

"At first I looked at high-end stuff because I always thought I was doing a great thing for myself by buying those products. But in the high-end store I couldn't find anything, not anything, that didn't have the trigger ingredients."

She tried natural products, but still had a hard time finding products without added fragrance or essential oils. "If your skin is really irritated and inflamed, why put more stuff than you need on it?" She started to use her nose as a guide. "Suddenly I would open these bottles and notice it had a smell of stuff that makes you just think, why would I want to put that on my skin? It smells like a chemists' lab." It took Laura Jones a long time to find products that made her feel safe as well as good about herself.

"My bottom line became choosing products where I read the ingredients and knew what they were, or where companies would explain the ingredients they were using," she said. These days, Laura buys products from a few trusted companies and keeps them in one little bag. She hasn't opened the silver toolbox in years. "It's toxic and old now," said the former makeup diva. But she can't quite throw it away. "It's too emotional. I think I have to have a ceremony or something to say goodbye."

According to the *Skin Deep* report, 82% of products contain immune system toxicants linked to allergies or sensitization.[13]

- Many products contain diethanolamine (DEA) or triethanolamine (TEA) as wetting agents. If the products also contain nitrites, a chemical reaction can lead to the formation of carcinogenic nitrosamines. Not all products containing DEA or TEA contain nitrosamines, but some may. Other ingredients that pose similar hazards for nitrosamine contamination are 2-bromo-2-nitro-propane-1,3-diol and Padimate-O.

Contaminants linked to breast cancer include PAHs (polycyclic aromatic hydrocarbons) and 1,3-butadiene. PAHs may be found in petrolatum, also called petroleum jelly. The contaminant 1,3-butadiene is a potential impurity in butane (also called n-butane), a propellant used in aerosol personal care products.[11] An easier way to avoid harmful contaminants is to use *Skin Deep*'s advanced search function to locate products that do not contain known impurities.[12]

## Get a Whiff of This

From Britney Spears' Fantasy to JLo's Glow, the sleek bottles promise love, wealth and celebrity appeal. But what they won't tell you is what's on the inside: complex mixtures of up to hundreds of chemicals that are not listed on labels. Fragrance is considered a trade secret, so companies don't have to disclose their ingredients. Almost half the products in *Skin Deep* contain the generic term "fragrance." Even "unscented" products may have masking fragrances — chemicals used to cover up the odor of other chemicals.

Some hidden hazards that may be lurking within synthetic-chemical fragrances include:

- *Allergens.* Fragrances are considered to be among the top five known allergens, and are known to both cause asthma and trigger asthma attacks.[14]

- *Phthalates.* Product tests conducted by Consumer Reports in January 2007 found the phthalates DEP and DEHP in all eight of eight perfumes tested.[15] The *Not Too Pretty* report found phthalates in 72% of personal care products, including fragrance-containing shampoos, deodorants and hair gels. None of the products listed phthalates on the label.[16]

- *Sensitizers.* One in every 50 people may suffer immune system damage from fragrance and become sensitized, according to the EU's

Scientific Committee on Cosmetic Products and Non-food Products.[17] Once sensitized to an ingredient, a person can remain so for a lifetime, enduring allergic reactions with every subsequent exposure.

As far back as 1986, the US National Academy of Sciences identified fragrance ingredients as one of six categories of neurotoxins (chemicals

## Sick of Scents

People tell her fragrance is a personal choice, but Carolyn Wysocki doesn't buy it. "They used to say smoking was a personal choice too. But if someone is smoking next to you or wearing fragrance next to you, you don't have a choice," said the psychologist and mother of four. Carolyn was working at a hospital in 1991 when she started feeling ill: headaches, trouble breathing, teary eyes. At first she suspected her symptoms were related to the massive renovations under way at the hospital because she felt better when she left work. But soon, it didn't matter where she was — at home, out shopping — Carolyn felt sick. She was eventually diagnosed with Multiple Chemical Sensitivity (MCS), a condition in which people develop increasing physical reactions to chemicals and air pollutants.

"For me, sometimes it's unbelievable, I can go into a building and sense immediately from the air that this is not a healthy building," Carolyn explained. Toxic exposures can cause her to get symptoms ranging from minor headaches to full-blown asthma attacks, muscle aches, confusion and disorientation. For people with MCS, the world can be an entirely dangerous place. Carolyn wears a respirator and makes careful choices about where she goes. Recently she was invited to speak at a community event that was advertised as "fragrance free," but her co-presenter showed up "doused with cologne." Soon, Carolyn was having trouble thinking straight. "Fortunately, I always write down my presentations word for word, because I never know when this is going to happen." She notices some fragrances are far worse than others, but without knowing the ingredients it's not possible to identify problem brands. So she asks friends and family to avoid all fragrance-containing products, including laundry detergents, as well as pesticides and other common triggers. Though it has taken some time, they've been cooperative. "At first my son-in-law wouldn't give up the fertilizers," Carolyn said. "But he finally did give it up, and do you know when that happened — when he had kids." The family is now using all unscented products and has switched to organic food.

toxic to the brain) that should be thoroughly investigated so we might better understand the impact to human health.[18] But government and industry have been slow to demand or fund such research. The FDA has taken no action on a petition submitted to the agency in 1999 requesting fragrance components be listed on labels.[19]

## Glossed Over

Formaldehyde, toluene, phthalates, acetone, methylacrylates — nail treatments are among the most toxic products in the *Skin Deep* database. But despite the toxic nature of the products — and the large population of nail salon workers who use them on a daily basis — very little epidemiological or occupational health research has been conducted on this population of women, according to a 2007 analysis of studies by Women's Voices for the Earth, *Glossed Over*.[20]

The few studies that have been conducted indicate cause for concern. Occupational health studies show decreased attention and processing skills as well as increased asthma in nail salon workers compared to women who don't work in salons. Women of childbearing age are particularly vulnerable due to the greater risk of chemical exposures to developing babies.

A survey of nail technicians in Boston found considerable awareness among the workers that their occupation was affecting their health. A majority of the workers surveyed reported odors at work that made them feel bad, and they associated these odors with acrylic nail glues. Survey respondents also reported experiencing work-related headaches, skin problems and respiratory problems. Many of these technicians reported feeling better when they were away from work for a day or two.[22] The National Asian Pacific American Women's Forum reports that Asian-American nail workers often feel powerless to change their work environments, and resistant to reporting the situation to occupational health authorities.[23]

In 2005 there were more than 57,000 nail salons in the US, employing more than 380,000 licensed nail technicians — 95% of these workers are women, and 59% are women of color. The average age of the workers is 38.[21]

The *Glossed Over* report is available in both English and Vietnamese and recommends short-term solutions for reducing risk, such as ventilating work spaces and providing employees with safety information. In the long term, the report calls for national legislation to eliminate toxic ingredients from cosmetics and studies to determine the long-term effects of chronic exposures to nail-product chemicals.

## What You Don't Know ...

For all the bad actors, *Skin Deep* identified a bigger-picture problem with cosmetics safety: most ingredients in cosmetic products have not been assessed for safety at all. According to Jane Houlihan's analysis, just 11% of cosmetic ingredients have been reviewed by the industry's Cosmetic Ingredient Review panel — the only publicly accountable institution that screens cosmetics ingredients for safety in the US.

The *Skin Deep* analysis also revealed deep deficiencies in the industry's self-policing panel. The panel is "dominated by dermatologists and almost all their decisions are driven by consideration of skin irritation or sensitization," Jane observed. But the panel was not set up for analyzing long-term health effects such as cancer or reproductive problems linked to cosmetic chemicals; they didn't have the expertise, the time (they spent an average of about 1.5 hours debating the science for each ingredient, Jane found), or the criteria in place to do so. "The panel does not have a framework or a policy on what is safe enough to use in cosmetics, so they make decisions all over the board," Jane said. "Sometimes we even found that they approved 'safe as used' chemicals in concentrations that were higher than levels where they saw effects in laboratory studies." Even in cases where the panel had found ingredients to be unsafe, the industry was free to ignore the recommendations.

The big finding of *Skin Deep* according to Jane Houlihan is that "the US doesn't have a safety standard for cosmetics." The US Food and Drug

### What does "safe" mean?

The FDA requires cosmetics companies to "adequately substantiate safety" of products, or else carry a warning label that says the safety of the product has not been determined. But there are no protocols or definitions for what it means to "substantiate safety," no requirements for companies to demonstrate safety — and not surprisingly, no products carrying the warning label. In 2004, EWG petitioned the FDA to recall products that violated the recommendations of the industry's safety panel, clarify what it means for companies to "adequately substantiate safety," and investigate products containing the most toxic chemical ingredients. The FDA denied the petition on all counts; the agency said it did not have the authority to take action.[24]

Administration has no authority to require companies to demonstrate personal care products are safe before putting them on the market. Instead, the companies get to decide for themselves what's safe. And as Jane found, "some companies are making products that are safe enough to eat, while others choose to regularly use carcinogens or developmental toxins. There's no baseline for them to work from, so anything goes and it's their own discretion."

## Skin Deeper Still

With no safety framework and little government oversight, the cosmetics industry is operating in a virtual Wild West. And the West has gotten wilder still.

- *Nanoemulsions* in shampoo encapsulate active ingredients and carry them deeper into hair shafts.
- *Nanosomes* of Pro-Retinol A penetrate the skin's surface to soften wrinkles and reduce the appearance of fine neck creases.
- *Nanovectors* transport and concentrate active ingredients in the skin.

*Deeper, faster, further.* As if there weren't enough concerns about the toxicity of cosmetic chemicals, manufacturers are rushing to incorporate nanotechnology that uses particles 80,000 times smaller than the width of a human hair. Nanotechnology has been touted as the next revolution in cosmetics and packaging. However, nanoparticles, being so tiny, have the potential to penetrate unusually deeply into the skin and organs, causing exotic physical effects.

Animal studies show that some nanoparticles can penetrate cells and tissues, move through the body and brain and cause biochemical damage.[25] As one example, carbon fullerenes — also called buckyballs, and currently being used in some moisturizers — can cause brain damage in fish, and even low levels of exposure can be toxic to human liver cells.[26] The health impacts of nanomaterials in cosmetics and sunscreens remain largely unknown, pending completion of long-range studies that have only recently begun. But that's not stopping the cosmetics industry from leading the charge to incorporate the inadequately tested technology into products we put on our faces and in our hair.

"In one of the most dramatic failures of regulation since the introduction of asbestos, corporations around the world are rapidly introducing thousands of tons of nanomaterials into the environment and onto the faces and hands of hundreds of millions of people, despite the growing body of evidence indicating that nanomaterials can be toxic for humans and the environment," said a May 2006 report by Friends of the Earth.[27] The group filed the first-ever legal challenge on the potential health impacts of nanotechnology in a 2006 petition to the FDA, demanding that the agency monitor and regulate nanoparticles in cosmetics.

Hundreds of personal care products already contain nano-sized ingredients, and thousands more contain ingredients that are available in nano form but don't include information about particle size on the labels, according to a *Skin Deep* analysis. Since nano-sized ingredients are absorbed differently into the body, they require separate safety studies. But as Jane Houlihan noted, "Manufacturers seem to be following the pattern they established with conventional chemical ingredients — put poorly tested chemicals into personal care products and do the science later, if at all."

The by-now familiar debate about cosmetics safety played out in the press coverage of the Friends of the Earth petition, as illustrated in a *San Francisco Chronicle* story.[28] "I don't think there's anything to worry about," Dr. John Bailey from the cosmetics industry trade association told the *Chronicle*. "All of the safety questions have been answered" in previous studies, he said. FDA spokeswoman Susan Cruzan said the agency has no evidence that nanoparticles in products pose hazards. Revlon and L'Oréal did not respond to the reporter's calls seeking comment. Estée Lauder spokeswoman Janet Bartucci said the company would review the Friends of the Earth report, and gave assurances that "consumer safety has always been a top priority at the Estée Lauder Companies." Lisa Archer from Friends of the Earth said she thinks corporations should "stop treating their customers like guinea pigs" by putting nanoparticles into personal care products before the materials are proven safe.

In the absence of federal regulations, some cities are trying to get a handle on the situation. Berkeley, California became the first city to regulate nanotechnology in December 2006, and other cities may follow suit. Under the Berkeley law, companies and research labs that make or use nanoparticles must disclose that fact to the city government and provide information about known health or safety risks.

## What Should I Buy?

"Just tell me which ingredients to avoid." It's the most common reaction people have upon hearing about the toxic cosmetics problem. Naturally, everyone wants the quick fix, the easy shopping list. But unfortunately, it doesn't exist. "The list of chemicals we know are toxic or contaminated is already too long for anyone to do an easy label check at the store," according to Alex Gorman, director of science and research at Women's Voices for the Earth. "And there are so many that should be on the list purely because we don't know anything about them. I wish I had more advice on this because I've struggled with it before and have never come up with a satisfying answer for folks asking the question." The ultimate answer, she said, is changing the law to require cosmetics companies to use the safest ingredients possible.

Until then, consumers can make more educated choices by using the *Skin Deep* database — and many are. The database gets about one million product searches per month. With its 2007 update, *Skin Deep* now offers brand-by-brand comparisons of more than 25,000 products, about one third of the market. "It's been such a great tool," Jane Houlihan said. "People use it to shop. Companies are using it to reformulate." She never could have guessed on the plane to California that her database would be such a lightning rod — nor did she know it would be a never-ending project.

"We'll be updating it every year," Jane said, "always pulling the latest toxicity databases, always adding more products." The staff at EWG — now including a chemist and medical doctor — continue to plug in new information, guided by a simple vision that is not so simple to carry out in the real world: "I want to walk into any store, anywhere, and buy any product without having to worry if it's safe for my wife and kids," said staffer Sean Gray.

Getting there will take more than a database. *Skin Deep* is "the beginnings of something empowering," said EWG staffer Hema Subramanian. "But how impossible is it for a mom with three kids on her arm to try to look everything up on a database and remember ingredients in the store? How do you make good choices without enough information out there?" Her experience with *Skin Deep* has made her a true believer in the need to reform government policies. "This is too overwhelming for a staff of five in a non-profit with a $3 million budget," she said. "There's too much responsibility placed outside of government. Companies need to be required to do more work on the front end to make products safer."

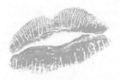

# 5

# Beauty Myth Busters

*For centuries, Japanese women have known a secret, the secret of beautiful skin. Prepare to discover the secret of SK-II for yourself. Many years ago, a Japanese monk noticed that the workers in a sake brewery had extraordinarily smooth hands. He was determined to discover why. After many experiments, he discovered a liquid that seemed to defy aging ...*

— *Advertisement for the premium brand
of SK-II skin care products*[1]

More recently Chinese authorities made a discovery of their own about SK-II products: the high-end skin whitening cream and powders contained the toxic heavy metals chromium and neodymium. "Hundreds of angry Chinese women have taken to the streets of Shanghai demanding refunds for US-Japanese cosmetics after authorities detected banned chemicals in some of the products," reported the *Agence France Presse* in September 2006. "Security guards were called in Thursday to control a crowd of about 300 people, infuriated over being made to wait over promised refunds for the affected SK-II cosmetics owned by US consumer products giant Procter and Gamble."[2]

P&G temporarily suspended sales of the SK-II line and closed sales counters across China after "security incidents" broke out between employees and customers and a furious mob smashed a glass door at the company's Shanghai branch.[3] Thousands of consumers demanded refunds of the elite brand that sells for more than $100 a bottle. It was a dramatic interruption in the otherwise relatively smooth and recent entry of multinational cosmetics corporations into the world's largest market.

The heavy metals chromium and neodymium, which can cause eczema and allergic dermatitis, are banned from cosmetics in China, although there are few other restrictions on personal care products. Procter & Gamble said the metals exist naturally, were not intentionally added to SK-II products and were safe at the low levels found in the products. In October, Chinese authorities announced the trace levels of metals would not harm consumers with normal use of the products, and by December SK-II products were slowly making their way back onto stores shelves.

Back at P&G company headquarters in the US, the episode presented no apparent difficulties. "The interruption is not expected to affect P&G's financial results," reported the *Cincinnati Enquirer*, in the city where the company's headquarters are based. "Sales in mainland China are only about 7% of global SK-II sales, and Procter said it removed SK-II from shelves simply to remove its products from the controversy until they were declared safe. China is P&G's fastest-growing market, with beauty-care products making up the bulk of the company's more than $2 billion in sales there."[4]

## White Hot

Skin whitening is all the rage in Asian countries like the Philippines, where the most popular actresses are light skinned, thin-nosed and appear in the ads for products that promise pale skin. "We're bombarded with advertisements like that every day. Every beauty product in the Philippines has a lightening aspect. Even lipstick promises to make dark upper lips more pink," said Anne Larracas from Quezon City near Manila.

Products in the category called "skin fading/skin lighteners" are among the most toxic cosmetics in the *Skin Deep* database. Many contain hydroquinone, which works as a skin lightener by decreasing the production of melanin pigments in the skin. The chemical — a confirmed animal carcinogen that is toxic to the skin, brain, immune system and reproductive system — is banned in the European Union but allowed in products sold in the US in concentrations of up to 2%. The US Cosmetic Ingredient Review panel warns the chemical is unsafe for use in products left on the skin, but the recommendation is sometimes ignored. Physicians Complex Skin Bleaching Cream with 2% hydroquinone, for example, advises consumers to "Apply to clean skin twice daily. Desired results are achieved with consistent use of this product." The product, made by CosMed, contains a dozen problematic ingredients, including three chemicals with potential to increase skin cancer risk by intensifying UV exposures in deep skin layers. "Application of Physicians Complex® sunblock SPF #30 is mandatory on a daily basis," advises the package.[5]

In the Philippines, where there are no regulated limits, some products, such as the popular Maxi Peel by Splash Corporation, contain 4% hydroquinone. Anne Larracas has friends who use such products, and she said the effects are startling. "When you first use it, as fast as three days, the skin starts to peel and it gets really red. Then the skin gets taut, you can see the veins because it peels too much, and the peeling doesn't stop. The skin gets lighter and lighter and thinner and thinner. Then the face starts to get light and white, but the neck is still dark, so it looks like there is a permanent foundation." Many women don't know they are supposed to also use sunscreen, Anne said. "It's so sad. I don't know why girls would like to whiten their skin."

According to dermatologists, skin color is genetic and no chemical can permanently lighten skin — although hydroquinone can produce temporary whitening effects, as can the heavy metals chromium and mercury, both of which have been detected in skin whitening creams sold in Asia. After the SK-II incident in China, media organizations in Hong Kong tested a range of skin whitening creams and reportedly found chromium in products made by Clinique, Estée Lauder, Christian Dior, Max Factor, Lancôme and Shiseido.[6] Mercury has also been detected in several products made in China and Taiwan. When a patient turned up in his office with mercury poisoning, Dr. Christopher Lam, chair at the department of chemical pathology at Hong Kong's Prince of Wales Hospital, examined her skin whitening cream and found mercury levels 65,000 times higher than amounts allowed in the US. Follow-up product tests conducted by Lam found mercury in eight of 38 skin whitening creams made in China and Taiwan. Some of the products were labeled "mercury free."[7]

Nevertheless, the "thriving *bihaku* (white beauty) boom remains one of the most significant driving forces for overall growth as manufacturers cater to the Asian preference for a fair complexion," reported *Euromonitor*. "According to leading industrial sources, up to 60% of Japanese women use skin whitening products in their daily regime, presenting manufacturers with a strong opportunity for continued growth." The major players have sought to maximize sales by offering "complete skin whitening regimes, comprising not only of moisturizers, but also cleansers, toners, day and night nourishers and even facial cleansing wipes." [8]

Sales are particularly promising in China, which has recorded double digit increases in recent years. The country is now the second largest market by volume for Procter & Gamble, and will someday be first if Daniela Riccardi, president of P&G Greater China, has her way. "Maybe it will take 10 years, but my staff, my company and I are very clear that it will eventually happen," the P&G executive told the *China Daily*. "Now our strategies are designed to touch as many customers in China as possible, step by step," Riccardi said. "Our future objective is to try to reach towns and villages where there are hundreds of millions of people." [9]

Not everyone is thrilled with the market potential. "I'm so pissed about this whitening stuff. It's everywhere," said Anne Larracas from the Philippines. "Every actress we have is light skinned, so when you're a *monena* like me, dark skinned, you have to use whitening products to become famous." Her cousin, a plastic surgeon, keeps teasing her to get a nose job. "The beauty stuff is symbolic of how we've been brainwashed about Western culture. It's the best thing to look Caucasian and blonde, with pretty light skin. And it's not just about beauty products, it's about clothes, iPods, books, TV shows, everything," Anne said. "What needs to happen is that we have to reconnect with who we really are."

## Mirror, Mirror on the Wall

Ken Harris admits to feeling a bit guilty about what he does for a living. As a "digital photo retoucher," he airbrushes fashion photos of the glamorous models who broadcast idealized images of beauty around the world. We know, of course, about the airbrushing. Still, it's surprising to see Harris in action in Jesse Epstein's award-winning documentary film *Wet Dreams and False Images*. [10] In the film, Harris demonstrated how he changes skin color, reshapes body parts and shaves pounds off models.

"Almost always the first thing I'll do is fix the nose," Harris explained, zipping the computer mouse over a photo. "Every picture has been worked on some 20 or 30 rounds going back and forth between the retouchers and the client and the agency. They're perfected to death," he said. "I don't see these photographs as being authentic or real. I see them as being mechanical and inhuman."

Digital retoucher Dominic Demasi demonstrated in the film how he reworked a photo of actress Halle Berry to remove pockmarks, change her skin tone to match her makeup and even shave down her knuckles to make them "seem less obtrusive." Product manufacturers are "not going to keep something that looks flawed or natural. They're not concerned with natural. They're concerned with selling their product," Demasi explained. "If it looks like it hasn't been touched at all, I've been successful."

The reshaped bodies, the smoothed-out wrinkles, "all that is there to alter your mind, to alter your conception of what physical beauty is ... and what the means of attaining it are," Harris said. "In that the central point of retouching is to enforce an unrealizable standard of beauty, I suspect of myself some sort of covert obscure misogyny, because I'm really screwing with people's sense of identity and self-worth by doing this." But, he said, he gets paid really well.

## The Straight Story

Felicia Eaves was eight when she started with the hair relaxers. Like many African-American girls, her hair was thick and tangled easily, causing many frustrating sessions under the brush. So twice weekly she used hair relaxer and styling aides — pomade or hair grease, as Felicia calls it, which kept her hair from drying out.

Of all the products in *Skin Deep*, those that change the shape and color of hair, such as relaxers, perms and dyes — along with nail products and skin lighteners — have the most toxic ingredients. The conditioners marketed to African-American women can also be problematic. "Instantly repair dry and damaged hair" is a typical marketing claim on hair products containing placenta, the nourishing fetal organ expelled after birth. Placenta products supposedly make hair stronger and more manageable, but they can also contain estrogenic hormones that are linked to early puberty and breast cancer. Some scientists believe that early and lifelong exposure to hormone-containing personal care products may be partly to blame for the high rates of breast cancer in young African-American women.[11]

It's not just the type of products used by African-American women that raises concern, but also the frequency of use. As Felicia Eaves, an organizer for Women's Voices for the Earth, explained, "We use more beauty products than other women, way more." According to market surveys, African-American women are more likely to take bubble baths, get facials and manicures, use scented products, wear lipstick and use bath additives than women of other ethnic groups. Nine out of ten African-American women use health and beauty products to express their individuality, compared to just over half of general market women. Though they comprise just 12% of the US population, African-American women account for 21% of all hair care expenditures.[12] Part of the reason, Felicia believes, is a special love affair with beauty products that stems from African heritage. The Egyptians were the first to discover and use cosmetics for the purposes of adornment some 6,000 years ago, and the bath ritual has always been an important part of African culture. "So I would say that we are subconsciously remembering what it was like to be in the motherland," said Felicia.

But another part of it, according to Felicia, is "the whole legacy of racism, the feeling that you need to look a certain way to be accepted in this society. The Eurocentric ideal of beauty in this country has really done a psychological job on African Americans. Every actress has a weave, even Oprah. Nobody is wearing their natural hair anymore." Traditional locks and afros are referred to as "extreme hair styles" in the popular culture, and young girls get the clear message about what's acceptable. Felicia has heard of girls as young as five getting weaves or extensions — these can be done naturally, but some involve glues and require acetone- or formaldehyde-based removers to get them off.

Felicia takes it back to "the whole crazy reason women do all this stuff to our bodies in the first place, because of a lack of self-esteem and a need to feel accepted. And it's not just Black women, it's all women." But there's a special pressure on Black women. "Throughout the history of slavery, Black women and men were used as a commodity, and because our look was so different, it was a point to ostracize us. There is this pressure that you have to look a certain way to be accepted. The way I look is still not quite as accepted as the way a White woman looks," Felicia said. "So part of it is about wanting to project a nice-looking image, but it also harkens back to how we've been perceived in this country, as different and other. We tend to want to be very careful about the way we're perceived with looks and hygiene."

In her view, women should be able to do whatever they want for a beauty routine without having to worry about toxic chemicals. "I like wearing makeup; I do get a lift from it. I like trying new colors and matching them with my outfits," Felicia said. "Women should be able to get that lift, but not at the expense of their health. The onus is on the manufacturers to make products that are safe."

## Paint Me Poison

As dark-skinned women dreamed of "white beauty," I was booking appointments at the tanning beds and lying for hours on end under the sun. The mineral oils and suntan lotions that promised bronze beauty littered my highschool vanity table along with dozens of jars, tubes and wands that covered up my anxieties. For me it was all about the Christie Brinkley fantasy — her flawless skin, that perfect nose! I studied the contours of the supermodel's face, scrutinized my profile, agonized; filled my little makeup bag with the tempting tropical hues that offered up the easy breezy Cover Girl dream.

Applying new knowledge to old habits, I take a trip back in time to see what secrets I can discover about my frequent forays to the Osco Drug aisle of hope. I typed my teen beauty routine into the *Skin Deep* database. The five shower products, liquid foundation, Clean Pressed Powder and Cheekers Blush; the Perfect Blend Eye Pencil, Expert Wear Shadows and Marathon Mascara, topped off with the daily cloud of Aqua Net Extra Super Hold. I counted 19 products in all — 230 chemicals, according to *Skin Deep*,[13] most of them applied to my body before I even left the house to catch the bus to Lynn Classical High. That's well above the average person's estimated daily exposure to cosmetic chemicals. Well, as I said, it was an obsession.

The first thing I notice is: so much for truth in advertising. Healing Garden Mintherapy Moisturizing Body Lotion by Coty Inc. gets the highest toxicity score of all the products on my list — a 4.1 (5 is the highest). Suave Lavender "Naturals" Shampoo and Conditioner by Unilever have 17 problematic ingredients between them. *Skin Deep* tells me: 81 of the chemical ingredients in my former daily routine raise health concerns. Some highlights:

- 22 daily doses of parabens, along with four other suspected hormone-disrupting chemicals.
- 17 hits of chemicals with limited or mixed evidence of carcinogenicity. One ingredient, petroleum distillates in my Cover Girl Marathon Waterproof Mascara, is banned in the European Union.
- 17 applications of penetration enhancers, which can draw the other chemicals more deeply into my body.
- 15 doses of chemicals that persist in the body or accumulate up the food chain.
- 15 products with fragrance — an unspecified mix of chemicals likely to contain phthalates and allergens.
- Less than half the ingredients in my products have been assessed for safety.

My head is spinning. I feel like Alice who fell down the rabbit hole. Down, down, down, until thump she goes into a long dark hallway with big keys and tiny locks. What does it all really mean? What does it mean, for instance, that the triethanolamine (or TEA) in my Ban de Soleil sunscreen, Healing Garden body lotion and Cover Girl "clean liquid" makeup has "limited evidence of carcinogenicity"? I delve deeper in the database and find that the chemical (spelled 32 different ways on product labels) forms carcinogenic nitrosamine compounds if mixed with other ingredients that act as nitrosating agents. It is also a skin sensitizer and possibly toxic to the lungs and brain.

I keep searching online and turn up a Material Safety Data Sheet on triethanolamine.[14] "Warning! Harmful if swallowed, causes skin irritation and severe eye irritation," says the emergency overview. The chemical has a moderate health rating, a slight rating for flammability and reactivity, and a severe contact rating. Goggles, gloves and lab coat are recommended in the lab. "Repeated ingestion has caused kidney and liver damage in animals." Doesn't sound so good; all sources agree the chemical has hazardous properties. But let's get real, there's probably only a tiny bit of TEA in my face makeup. What's the actual risk to my health?

The Mad Hatter appears, clipboard in hand, to explain that in order to calculate a risk assessment, one must review the science to determine the chemical hazard, and then estimate how much of the chemical a person is exposed to: Risk = Hazard + Exposure. These are the type of calculations the Cosmetic Ingredient Review panel used to review TEA and determine the chemical is "safe with qualifications" in cosmetics, with concentration limits for leave-on-the-skin products. So, assuming the companies stuck to the concentration limits, I am safe?

Not so fast. Triethanolamine, I learned in my research, is also used in floor polish, pool cleaners, rug cleaners, laundry detergent, toilet bowl cleaners and other products I may have been exposed to on the day I used the three beauty products. The risk assessment didn't account for that. It also can't tell me what happens when TEA is mixed in combination with the 16 other potential carcinogens, two dozen endocrine disruptors and other toxic substances in my daily routine. Few, if any, of the chemicals in my cosmetics have been tested in mixtures to understand the long-term health impacts of chronic use over time. And since most risk assessments are calculated to figure risk for a typical 160-pound male, it may not accurately account for the impact on a teenage girl whose breasts and body were developing when the products were applied. Hmmm. All very curious.

So what's young Alice to do? As the landscape tilts and twirls, a picture comes clear: it is exactly the complicating factors of it — the dozens of toxic chemicals, combined into mixtures that have never been assessed for safety — that are the truest truth of all. Nobody can tell me what impact these daily chemical cocktails had on my body. Now, as the Lewis Carroll story goes, wise young Alice already knew to check the bottle to see if it was marked "poison" — "for she had read several nice little stories about children who had got burnt, and eaten up by wild beasts, and other unpleasant things, all because they *would* not remember the simple rules their friends had taught them: such as, that a red-hot poker will burn you if you hold it too long and that, if you cut your finger very deeply with a knife, it usually bleeds; and she had never forgotten that, if you drink much from a bottle marked 'poison,' it is almost certain to disagree with you, sooner or later." [15] But, of course, none of the 19 bottles and tubes on my vanity table carried such a warning.

Still, it's just a little bit of poison, right? What's the harm in that? After all, I am healthy, energetic and relatively intact two decades after my teen-beauty-queen phase. Many women and men who have enough disposable income to buy beauty products will go on to live long, happy and healthy lives. There are plenty of other things to worry about as the newspaper reminds me: terrorism, war, global warming and murders in nearby Oakland. All true.

But I also can't help wondering about the two benign lumps in my body that required surgical removal and my four-year struggle with infertility in my 20s. I asked my doctor — a brilliantly talented surgeon who has removed the thyroids of thousands of young women in the Massachusetts area — why I developed a lump on my thyroid (the size of a lemon, it turned out) and why so many other young women are getting them too. Could mine have had anything to do with the fact that I grew up a mile from the largest polluting trash-burning facility in the state? "Hmmm," he replied, giving me a funny look. "Don't know. Nobody has ever asked me that before. We don't know why thyroid lumps happen, they just do." It was the same story with the infertility. After many expensive tests, the doctors declared unknown cause and suggested I try the pharmaceutical drug Clomid. The doctors will never be able to tell me if environmental factors — pollution from the RESCO incinerator in nearby Saugus, the black smokestacks of the Salem oil refineries or the chemical exposures in my childhood home — contributed to my health issues.

A friend from Iran reports that her family bugs her to get a nose job whenever she goes home — everyone in Tehran is doing it, even the men. A friend in South Carolina reports that several of her neighbors are getting breast implants. A friend from India remembers being pressured to use "fair and lovely" skin lightener as a little girl. Visit NotJustaPrettyFace.org to join an online discussion about busting the beauty myth.

The way I see it, even the smokestacks aren't separate from the Healing Garden Mintherapy lotion and its 4.1 toxicity score — coming as it does from oil-derived petrochemicals, and ending up as it often does (plastic case and all) burning up in waste incinerators located near working-class communities like Lynn. In the real world, my lungs breathe the air from the smokestacks and the fumes from the rug cleaner at the same time as my skin absorbs the toxic chemicals from the face lotion.

Back down in the rabbit hole, the most sensible sense of all came from the short e-mail I received from cosmetic chemist Bruce Akers when I asked his opinion about triethanolamine: "It is shitty and there are many better alternatives."

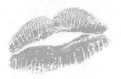

# 6

# *Pinkwashing*

Pinkwashing: a term used to describe the activities of companies and groups that position themselves as leaders in the struggle to eradicate breast cancer while engaging in practices that may be contributing to rising rates of the disease.

The bald woman in the pink T-shirt looks wistfully off into the distance in the ad in *Yoga Journal*. She is standing in a sea of pink hats and hopeful faces. *We can live without our hair,* the caption says. *We can live without our breasts. We cannot live without our hope for a cure.* I feel the anguish of this woman, recalling images that will never leave me: my grandmother doubled over on the chair with blood leaking from the bandage where her breast used to be; my terror when I first brushed across the lump in my own breast. I want to hug this bald woman in the ad and cry with her. But I also want to shout: *We should not have to live without our hair! We should not have to live without our breasts! Why is this happening?*

In just my lifetime, the risk of getting breast cancer for women living in the United States increased dramatically. More American women have died of breast cancer in the last 20 years than the number of Americans killed in World War I, World War II, the Korean War and the Vietnam War combined. Once a disease almost exclusive to postmenopausal women, breast cancer now strikes women in their 20s and 30s — especially young African-American women — and it is the second leading cause of death (after heart disease) in American women ages 25–54. What's going on?

More than half of all breast cancer cases can't be explained by any of the known risk factors, such as genetics, diet or reproductive history. Growing evidence indicates that the explanation lies in the environment around us: in the carcinogens and hormone-disrupting chemicals women are routinely exposed to throughout our lives. The patterns of breast cancer indicate the importance of environmental factors. Breast cancer rates are much higher in industrialized countries, such as North America and northern Europe, than in developing countries. People who move to industrialized countries from countries with lower breast cancer rates soon develop the higher rates of their new country.[1]

The increase in breast cancer also parallels the proliferation of man-made chemicals since World War II. Many of these chemicals persist in the environment, accumulate in body fat and can remain in breast tissue for decades. Some have been shown to induce mammary tumors in animals, while others disrupt the delicate hormonal balance in the body. "Compelling scientific evidence points to some of the 100,000 synthetic chemicals in use today as contributing to the development of breast cancer, either by altering hormone function or gene expression," according to *State of the Evidence 2006: What Is the Connection between the Environment and Breast Cancer?*, a report that summarizes more than 350 studies on the environmental links to breast cancer. The report, published by the Breast Cancer Fund and Breast Cancer Action and peer-reviewed by leading scientists, also identifies radiation exposure, such as nuclear radiation and X-rays, as the "longest-established environmental cause of breast cancer."[2]

Among chemicals of concern, suspicion focuses on substances that act like estrogen in the body. There is broad agreement in the scientific community that higher exposure to estrogens over a woman's lifetime leads to a higher risk of developing breast cancer. For example, girls who menstruate before age 12 are 50% more likely to develop breast cancer than girls who menstruate after age 16, in part because of the increased lifetime exposure to estrogen. Early breast development is also clearly associated with an increased breast cancer risk. Both these phenomena — earlier onset menarche and earlier breast development — are occurring with disturbing regularity in US girls, and even more dramatically in African-American girls, according to a 2007 report by biologist Sandra Steingraber, PhD, distinguished visiting scholar at Ithaca College in New York. Several factors may hasten the onset of puberty in girls, including low birth weight and premature birth, obesity and environmental exposures to endocrine-disrupting chemicals, Dr. Steingraber reported.[3]

The evidence suggests that the metaphor of the reproductive system as a "biological clock" — a fixed entity insensitive to environmental input — is misleading. "Puberty is less like a clock and more like a musical performance, with our bodies as the keyboards and the environment

## Reducing Carcinogens

In May 2007, the Silent Spring Institute and Susan B. Komen for the Cure released the most comprehensive scientific review of mammary carcinogens to date. The report identified 216 chemicals that cause breast cancer in animals, including industrial solvents, pesticides, dyes, cosmetics ingredients, hormones and pharmaceuticals.

"Overall, exposure to mammary gland carcinogens is widespread," the researchers wrote in a special supplement to the journal *Cancer*. "These compounds are widely detected in human tissues and in environments, such as homes, where women spend time."

Some of the most widespread mammary carcinogens include:

- 1,4-dioxane — found in detergents, shampoos, soaps
- 1,3-butadiene — common air pollutant; found in vehicle exhaust
- Perfluorooctanoic acid — used in manufacture of Teflon
- Vinyl chloride — used to make PVC/vinyl plastic
- PAHs — from diesel and gasoline exhaust
- PCBs — electrical transformers; banned but still in environment
- Atrazine — a herbicide widely used in the US, but banned in Europe

Because breast cancer is so common and the exposure to the chemicals so widespread, "the public health impacts of reducing exposures would be profound even if the true relative risks are modest," the researchers wrote. "If even a small percentage is due to preventable environmental factors, modifying these factors would spare thousands of women." [4]

(both internal and external) as the hands of the pianist," Dr. Steingraber said. "Our bodies are the mediums for a much larger message; as we change that message, we change ourselves."

Another disturbing trend that has researchers looking to environmental explanations is the rising incidence of breast cancer in young African-American women. Compared with women of their grandmothers'

According to *State of the Evidence*, synthetic chemicals that can mimic estrogen or disrupt hormones in the body include:

- Bisphenol A — a component of polycarbonate plastic (#7), used in baby bottles and water coolers
- Parabens — used as preservatives in a range of cosmetics
- Phthalates — used in personal care products and vinyl plastic
- Placental extract — used in hair products marketed primarily to African-American women

The vast majority of chemicals have not been tested for hormone-disrupting effects or their potential to cause breast tumors.[5]

# The Good News

After a decades-long increase, breast cancer rates in the US have been falling in recent years. An analysis of statistics by researchers at the University of Texas M.D. Anderson Cancer Center found that the most common form of breast cancer, estrogen positive tumors, declined a startling 15% in women ages 50–69 between 2002 and 2003 — the first significant drop in breast cancer rates in a quarter century. The researchers believe the reason is that millions of women abandoned hormone replacement therapy after a large federally funded study reported that women who regularly took the menopause drug Prempro (a combination of estrogen and progestins) were more likely to develop heart problems and breast cancer. Soon after the findings emerged, many women stopped using the hormones and breast cancer rates began falling, the statistics show.[6] The findings raise the question: could reducing exposure to other sources of external synthetic estrogens further reduce breast cancer rates?

generation, African-American women have a 41% greater rate of invasive breast cancer and White women have a 21% greater rate, according to a 2006 analysis by researchers at the University of Pittsburgh Cancer Institute Center for Environmental Oncology and the Graduate School of Public Health.[7] African-American women under 40 have a higher incidence of breast cancer than White women in this age group, and they are more likely to die of the disease at any age. The known risk factors can't explain the ethnic variations, the researchers said.

But the researchers point to something they believe may explain the difference: hormone-containing personal care products. "We hypothesize that the use of estrogen and other hormone-containing personal care products in young African-American women accounts, in part, for their increased risk of breast cancer prior to menopause, by subjecting breast buds to elevated estrogen exposure during critical windows of vulnerability in utero and in early life," the researchers wrote in the scientific journal *Medical Hypotheses.*[8]

The paper notes that African-American females are more likely than whites to experience early sexual maturity, and they are also more likely to use hormone-containing personal care products, such as hair pomades and conditioners with placental extracts. "Some of these compounds are widely used in the African-American community throughout life, starting at very young ages," said senior investigator Devra Davis, PhD, director of the UPCI Center for Environmental Oncology. The paper cites several reports linking hormone-containing personal care products to premature sexual development. In one case, Black toddlers began to develop breasts and pubic hair when their parents applied hair pomades to their scalps. "When they stopped using these products, the breasts went away," Dr. Davis said. "Now anything that can make breasts grow in an infant has got to be problematic."[9]

More research is needed to verify or refute a link between personal care products and breast cancer, although the paper notes that research is hampered by the lack of publicly available information about hormone-mimicking compounds in personal care products. The researchers called on cosmetics companies to disclose their use of hormonally active ingredients so research can move forward. But, said Dr. Devra Davis, "We don't just want to study the problem, we want to make the problem go away." She believes there is enough evidence to justify removing questionable compounds now. "As scientists, we'll never know enough. It's inherent

in science that there is uncertainty. But just because something is complicated doesn't mean we can't understand it," Dr. Davis said. "It comes down
to, how much proof do we need? If we insist that the only proof we'll
accept is dead bodies and sick people, than we are dooming our kids to
getting sick before we can take action to protect them." Dr. Davis said
she is particularly concerned about products containing placenta, parabens
preservatives, phthalates, formaldehyde preservatives and heavy metals
as well as products marketed to young children that are contaminated with
carcinogenic impurities. Her advice to women is "simpler is better" —
use fewer products, choose products with fewer synthetic or unknown
ingredients, and avoid hormonally active ingredients when possible.

The news about environmental links to breast cancer is, ultimately,
hopeful news: it means we can take collective action to reduce risk. "We
can't change our parents, but we can change our environment. We can
change, for God's sake, the ingredients in nail polish," said Dr. Sandra
Steingraber. The *State of the Evidence 2006* report called for new government policies that require companies to phase out harmful chemicals
and favor safer alternatives, and new research agendas that focus on the
preventable causes of breast cancer.[10] "We need to eliminate, as much as
possible, human exposures to all substances or agents known or suspected of contributing to the disease process," said Jeanne Rizzo, RN,
executive director of the Breast Cancer Fund. What it's really going to
take to reduce breast cancer, she said, is "a revolution in thinking on the
parts of government and the private sector."

## Pink It Up

What we find in the mainstream culture instead is a revolution in shopping. We can "shower for the cure" with pink ribbon gel, dust our cheeks
with "Hint of a Cure" blush and "Kiss Good Bye to Breast Cancer" with
Avon lipstick. We can "test drive a BMW for the cure," buy an iPod
"Case for a Cause" and "save lids to save lives" with Yoplait yogurt —
though you'd have to eat three yogurts a day for four months to raise
$36 for the cause, points out the nonprofit group Breast Cancer Action
on their "Think Before You Pink" website.[11] The site urges consumers
to ask critical questions about pink-ribbon products and promotions,
such as: How much money goes to the cause? What is it supporting?
What is the company doing to ensure its products don't contribute to
breast cancer?

Some pink-ribbon promoters would rather not confront such questions. For instance, the cosmetics companies' high-profile efforts to raise money for the cause include Revlon's 5K Run/Walk and the Estée Lauder Companies' Annual Breast Cancer Awareness Campaign — billed as "the Power of a Pink Promise." Yet both companies were singled out in the 2005 *Skin Deep* report, which included a list of "Top 20 Brands of Concern" based on toxicity. Revlon's Ultima II and the Estée Lauder brand were 8 and 9 on the list, respectively.[12] Both companies make products that contain suspected carcinogens and hormone-disrupting chemicals, as does Avon, which claims to be the largest corporate supporter of the breast cancer cause in the US.[13] Through their trade association, the Cosmetic, Toiletry, and Fragrance Association, the companies opposed a California bill that would require cosmetics companies to disclose their use of chemicals linked to cancer or birth defects.[14] And none of the three companies has signed the Compact for Safe Cosmetics, a pledge to remove hazardous chemicals and replace them with safer alternatives.

All of this outrages Jeanne Rizzo of the Breast Cancer Fund. "If they're concerned about the cause and prevention side of the disease — and I don't know how they could not be — Estée Lauder, Revlon and Avon ought to be in the leadership on this issue, not having to be pushed on it," Rizzo said. "When new knowledge comes to you that your product contains problematic ingredients, if you were authentic in your support for breast cancer, you would be vigilant in addressing that." Instead, the pink-ribbon cosmetics companies defend their use of hazardous chemicals ("it's just a little bit") and fight to keep their industry unregulated. "It points out a lack of sincerity about the issue. They chose breast cancer because it's women and that's their market."

It's not that having an iconic symbol for a disease is a bad idea, Rizzo points out. For many women, wearing the pink ribbon and participating in community events is important and validating. But the pink ribbon, with its carefully contrived message about "awareness" and "hoping for the cure," also serves to distract from a deeper public discussion about preventable causes of breast cancer. "It is the very blandness of breast cancer, at least in mainstream perceptions, that makes it an attractive object of corporate charity and a way for companies to brand themselves friends of the middle-aged female market," wrote author Barbara Ehrenreich.[15] Companies want to support breast cancer because "breast cancer is safe," said Carol Cone, who helped kick off "cause marketing" in the 1980s with research showing that, given the same cost and quality, more than half of consumers would switch from a particular brand to one associated with a good cause.[16] With breast cancer "there was no concern that you might actually turn off your audience because of the lifestyle or sexual connotations that AIDS has," Amy Langer, director of the National Alliance of Breast Cancer Organizations, told the *New York Times* in 1996. "That gives corporations a certain freedom and a certain relief in supporting the cause." [17] Or, as National Women's Health Network director Cindy Pearson put it: "Breast cancer provides a way of doing something for women, without being feminist." [18]

And there's the rub. With its focus on moving products, the pink ribbon excludes all notions of feminism, activism, corporate accountability or changing the status quo. Instead, the public conversation — and much of the research — narrows in on a set of topics that don't rain on the corporate cash parade. We hear a lot of hype about pharmaceutical solutions for breast cancer, but not much about prevention strategies such as cleaning up carcinogens in the environment. We hear that fewer women are dying of breast cancer, but there's little discussion about how many more women are *getting* the disease. We're told to take personal responsibility and make good lifestyle choices, such as eating right and exercising. But there's barely a whisper about industry's responsibility to reduce pollution and use precaution. Tugging the ends of the pink ribbon, one starts to unravel some reasons why.

## Raining Ribbons

The pink ribbon was originally neither pink nor was it intended to be used as a marketing tool. It was a peach ribbon developed in the early 1990s by Charlotte Haley, who watched her daughter, sister and grandmother suffer breast cancer. Angry and determined to start a grassroots movement, Charlotte sat down at her dining room table and crafted thousands of peach ribbons by hand. She bundled them into sets of five, each with a card that read: "The National Cancer Institute annual budget is $1.8 billion; only 5 percent goes for cancer prevention. Help us wake up our legislators and America by wearing this ribbon." She distributed the bundles at her local supermarket and wrote to Dear Abby and other prominent women to call attention to the campaign.[19]

At that time, breast cancer was just starting to come out of the closet, and a couple of major corporations had big plans. Estée Lauder and *Self* magazine teamed up to create the second annual Breast Cancer Awareness Month issue, and they envisioned a breast cancer ribbon displayed on cosmetics counters from coast to coast. But somebody already had a breast cancer ribbon, they were told. So they called up Charlotte Haley offering to partner with her and take her peach ribbon national. "She wanted nothing to do with us. Said we were too commercial," *Self* magazine editor Alexandra Penney explained to *MAMM* magazine.[20] For Charlotte, the ribbon was a tool to inspire women to become politically active, not to sell products. But her vision was not to be realized. Estée Lauder and *Self* really wanted that ribbon. Their lawyers advised them to choose another color. Pink, a life-affirming color known for its calming, quieting, stress-reducing effects, was the color chosen. "In focus groups and studies, pink came out as something that was warm, happy, pleasant and playful, which is everything that breast cancer is not for women who are living with the disease," commented Brenda Salgado of Breast Cancer Action. "So that's where the pink ribbon was born. And Charlotte Haley's peach ribbon just kind of disappeared, inundated under pink ribbons ever after."

## Cancer Inc.

Unraveling the ribbon further, one finds even more disturbing contents inside the pink package. "They make the chemicals, they run the treatment centers, and they're still looking for 'the cure' — no wonder they won't tell you about breast cancer prevention," begins the expose by Sharon Batt and Liza Gross in *Sierra* magazine.[21] It's the most straightforward way to put it.

The co-founder and major sponsor of Breast Cancer Awareness Month is AstraZeneca (formerly known as Zeneca), a British-based multinational giant that manufactures the cancer drug tamoxifen, the most widely prescribed breast cancer drug. Until 2000, the company was also a leading manufacturer of agricultural chemicals, including the carcinogenic pesticide acetochlor. When Zeneca created National Breast Cancer Awareness Month in 1985, it was owned by Imperial Chemical Industries, a multi-billion-dollar producer of pesticides, paper and plastics. The company was named in a 1990 lawsuit by the federal government for allegedly dumping DDT and PCBs into the Los Angeles and Long Beach harbors.[22] After buying up cancer clinics around the country, Zeneca merged with the Swedish pharmaceutical company Astra in 1999 to form AstraZeneca, the world's third largest drug company.

"This is a conflict of interest unparalleled in the history of American medicine," said Dr. Samuel Epstein, a professor of occupational and environmental medicine at the University of Illinois School of Public Health. "You've got a company that's a spin-off of one of the world's biggest manufacturers of carcinogenic chemicals, they've got control of breast cancer treatment, they've got control of the chemoprevention [studies], and now they have control of cancer treatment in eleven centers — which are clearly going to be prescribing the drugs they manufacture." [23]

They've also got control over the public message of National Breast Cancer Awareness Month, which focuses on early detection — in other words, find out if you've already got the disease. "The awareness is about getting your mammograms and getting pills," said Brenda Salgado. "It focuses all our attention on 'early detection' and 'cure,' which is important for women who currently have cancer, but it keeps us from the equally important effort of preventing women from getting the disease in the first place. It also avoids the critical questions the breast cancer epidemic raises. What is the connection between environmental toxins and breast cancer? And why has the incidence of breast cancer risen, despite the 'war on cancer' and all the money spent on research?"

The nation's largest breast cancer charities fall in line with similar messages about early detection and cure, and divert public attention away from prevention strategies in ways that are sometimes not so subtle. The American Cancer Society (ACS), for instance, is frequently quoted in the press urging cautious interpretation of evidence linking chemicals to disease. As one example: a July 2005 *New York Times* story entitled "Should You Worry About the Chemicals in Your Makeup?" quoted Dr. Michael Thun, head of epidemiology at ACS, questioning the science on phthalates. "There are real uncertainties about animal studies," Thun said.[24] However, expert panels at the US National Toxicology Program have said the animal studies on phthalates are likely to predict human reproductive health effects.[25]

ACS also dismissed a report by the California EPA, based on an exhaustive analysis of two decades of research, that second-hand smoke is linked to premenopausal breast cancer. According to Jeanne Rizzo of the Breast Cancer Fund, this is an indication of an institutionalized culture of resistance. "Not only is the American Cancer Society not taking leadership, there's a resistance," she said. "They are willing to look at alcohol, obesity, diet and genetics. But are they willing to look at what's making girls go into puberty earlier? Are they willing to look at the links between chemicals and cancer? Their focus is on cure. There's a normalization of cancer in that model when you don't look at causes of cancer. It's like saying you're going to get it — but we'll cure it."

## Look Good, Feel Better

We may get cancer, but at least we'll look good when we do.

"Give cancer the brush," says the ad for "Look Good ... Feel Better," the flagship cancer program of the Cosmetic, Toiletry, and Fragrance Association (CTFA).[26] The program offers free makeup to women recovering from cancer treatments — a generous gesture, yes, but also a bit jarring with its head-patting tone and focus on pushing products. "Experiencing skin, facial and nail changes during cancer treatment? You can still be yourself. Our make-over expertise will show you the way to look good ... feel better ... just follow the numbers below," instructs the website. When one follows the numbers — Step 1 "straightforward skin care" through Step 9 "nail care and polish" — one is overwhelmed with how-to tips for an elaborate makeover that recommends no less than 25 cosmetic products. Step 9, at least, recommends selecting a nail polish without formaldehyde, which "increases dryness and yellowing," according to the website. But it does not mention that formaldehyde is also a known carcinogen.

The program has its roots in a story about a depressed patient and her doctor, who contacted CTFA then-president Ed Kavanaugh asking for advice about overcoming appearance-related side effects. Ed made some calls and obtained free cosmetics and the services of a makeup artist. "Miraculously, the makeover transformed not just the woman's look, but her outlook as well. She immediately felt happier and less burdened, laughing for the first time in weeks. The doctor credited the makeover with improving her attitude and emotional approach toward her treatment," the website reports. "With such a profound result, the CTFA recognized the opportunity for its industry to help more women maintain self-esteem and face cancer treatment with greater confidence."

The American Cancer Society enthusiastically joined the effort along with the National Cosmetology Association, and "Look Good ... Feel Better" flourished across the nation, with programs now in all 50 states.

There is even a "Look Good ... Feel Better for Teens" program for cancer patients ages 13 to 17 — a growing demographic since childhood cancer rates have been increasing. The program addresses the needs of both boys and girls, and its interactive, information-packed website covers skin care, head coverings, makeup, fitness and nutrition, and offers "tips for dealing with friends, fatigue, activities, school, and looking your best through it all." [27]

## Not So Hot Trends

The normalization of cancer is everywhere. It's the kind of thing that, once you notice it, hits you in the gut every time, casting a dark shadow on messages that are supposed to be comforting and reassuring. The 60-year-old grandparents in the TV commercial play happily with their baby granddaughter on the backyard swing, thanks to medicine that keeps them from getting sick from chemotherapy. The *Parade* magazine story paints a happy scene of kids in a cancer-treatment center throwing "off chemo" parties, complete with cake and ice cream. The movie trailer shows a circle of sad-looking bald kids, prompting us to "hope for the cure."

Some people accused California lawmakers of "voting on emotion" when they approved a bill requiring cosmetics companies to disclose their use of chemicals linked to cancer. Yes, this *is* about emotion — it's about grief, and love too, those age-old human traits. "My 27-year-old nephew was just diagnosed with Stage 3 testicular cancer," Jeanne Rizzo told me at the end of our half-hour conversation about pink ribbons. "I want that kid cured," she said, her voice rising. "I don't care if they have to dump a superfund site down his veins. But I don't want my son and my other nephew to get it either. How can you ignore the prevention part of it?"

As the teen cancer programs remind us, cancer is everywhere and it's everyone's problem. Everyone needs to be part of the solution too — especially the wealthy corporations that brand themselves to breast cancer. "They have two responsible choices," Jeanne Rizzo said of the pink-ribbon-waving Avon, Revlon and Estée Lauder. "They can keep using crappy chemicals and find another cause to support. Or they can make an authentically valuable social contribution by refusing to buy carcinogens and hormone-disrupting chemicals from the chemical companies." Now that would be a truly powerful Pink Promise.

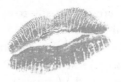

# 7

## *Because We're Worth It Too!*

Teenagers have a certain way of just cutting to the chase. "It's disgusting that women can get rid of our toxins by passing them on to our babies," said Jessica Assaf. Before she has that experience though, Jessica plans to go to college, become a pediatric oncologist and pressure the cosmetics industry to clean up its products. On a Saturday morning in February 2006, Jessica, Heather Gellert and about 20 of their peers from various high schools in Marin County, California, stood before a crowd of mostly other teens who had traveled here to learn how to organize safe cosmetics campaigns in their own schools. In just a year, the Marin girls had accomplished a head-spinning amount with their teen-led campaign.

Two by two, the teens approached the microphone and told their story as if it was nothing at all to stand in front of a roomful of people discussing science and politics on a Saturday morning. Watching them from the audience, I felt like I'd entered an alternate universe. I didn't even know what lobbying was when I was that age. Mine is a typical reaction. "People are just like wow. They're not used to teens sounding like this. They're not used to teens being as educated and as wise," explained Judi Shils, founder of the Marin Cancer Project, where Teens for Safe Cosmetics got their start. "They're all really pretty girls. They wear a lot of makeup; it's a big part of their lives. When they found out their favorite products were potentially toxic, they were furious. They wanted to rattle every cage they could."

A four-time Emmy Award–winning former television producer, Judi founded the Marin Cancer Project in 2002 after being inspired by a friend who had just completed treatment for a radical breast cancer. Marin County had the highest rates of breast cancer in the US, they learned at a county meeting. The rates had risen 60% in eight years, and nobody could explain why.[1] "Here we are in one of the richest counties in the world and there's no money for research? We're here talking about elevated cancer rates and we don't know why, and nothing is being done. I thought there had to be a better way to get a community to come together around these issues," Judi explained. So, after amassing 2,000 volunteers, they went door-to-door one day in November 2002 asking people to fill out a health survey and give a dollar for cancer research. Judi wasn't sure if residents would just slam their doors; instead, people wanted to talk and talk about their experiences with cancer. Before long the volunteers raised close to $150,000 to fund a research project to map cancer rates in the towns of Marin.[2]

After that Judi thought she'd move on to her next project, leaving the scientists to do their work, but in her own words "you step your foot into something and get wisdom and the support of the community, and you can't go away." She became interested in cosmetics after her teenage daughter Erin started filling up her little makeup bag. "We started going to supermarkets and looking at labels and seeing all these chemicals we can't pronounce and looking them up on the Internet," Judi said. They found *Skin Deep*, learned about the work of the Campaign for Safe Cosmetics and decided to try to get something going in Marin County. In January 2005, Judi and Erin invited local high school students to a forum they called Safe Cosmetics 101. When 85 girls showed up on a school night, Judi knew they were onto something. Cosmetics and personal care products are a lightning rod issue for teenagers, she realized. "It's one thing everybody does every day. We all wash our hair and brush our teeth and put on deodorant, and girls wear makeup. It's a metaphor for looking and thinking about every aspect of our lives."

The girls started to make changes right away. As Branson High School sophomore Jessica Assaf told me, "The first thing I did is that I went home and looked at my products and started looking at the ingredients.

I was using about 15 products a day. It really shocked me that I had no idea what I was putting on my body and what my friends and family were putting on their bodies." One by one, she switched to less-toxic products "starting with my deodorant because, if you think about it, especially for women, you're putting it right by your breasts." She joined the core group of about 20 girls who started meeting weekly after the forum to organize a teen cosmetics campaign. "The idea was that they had to do the work," Judi Shils explained. "We weren't going to sit there and tell them that products are bad and you should change them. They figured out what they had to figure out and found products that were better versions of whatever they were using. They did their due diligence and really worked hard at it."

The first thing the teens decided to do was survey their peers to find out which products were most popular. Then they researched the ingredients and talked about how to put that information back out into the community in ways that would empower people to make better decisions. They created a "picks and pans" list of toxic products and safer choices and made a giant wooden face to display the products. They got on TV with their face, wrote articles for local papers and put together a Safe Cosmetics Bill of Rights, which they presented to the Marin County Board of Supervisors.

"Each girl had her own strength and worked on what she felt the most strongly about," according to Judi Shils. The girls worked with an ad agency and design firm to create marketing materials and did their own research and media outreach. "The experiences they're having and the life skills they're learning, these girls are going to go on in their lives and do things that are unbelievable," Judi said. "If you can engage teens to really get involved in something they are passionate about, it becomes part of their daily lives, there's so much they can do to effect change that adults cannot."

## Beauty Queens Take on the Governator

"California Gov. Arnold Schwarzenegger is no girlie man — just ask him — but he does wear makeup," observed columnist Marjie Lundstrom in the *Sacramento Bee*.[3] "So will he, or won't he?" The question was on the minds of teenagers, actors and corporate CEOs alike: would the Republican governor sign or veto one of the most heavily lobbied bills of the 2005 legislative session? The California Safe Cosmetics Act of

2005, sponsored by Senator Carol Migden (D-San Francisco), would require cosmetics manufacturers to disclose to the state if they were using chemicals linked to cancer or birth defects. Despite heavy lobbying by the cosmetics industry, the bill known as SB 484 had passed the legislature with bipartisan support in a 43–35 vote in August of 2005. Now it was sitting on the governor's desk.

The story had all the makings of a great drama. "So here is our pro-business Republican governor with his tough-guy image, under pressure from teenage girls and beauty queens and fellow actors over beauty products — a Hollywood staple," Lundstrom described in the *Bee*. "So relentless was Migden in ensuring her bill's passage that she popped over to the floor of the Assembly during a vote and pushed a Republican member's 'yes' button. Meanwhile, the $35 billion industry unleashed its own big guns on the Capitol in what bill supporters saw as a 'David and Goliath' confrontation."

"The legislators had never seen anything like it," reported Janet Nudelman of the Breast Cancer Fund. "They were literally hiding because so many industry representatives were roaming the halls." Led by the industry trade group — the Cosmetic, Toiletry, and Fragrance Association (CTFA) — lobbyists swarmed the state capitol wearing matching "No on SB 484" pins. Mary Kay, Avon, Estée Lauder, L'Oréal, Neutrogena, Johnson & Johnson and other major companies lined up at legislative hearings to testify against the bill. According to state records, Procter & Gamble paid Sacramento lobbyists more than $260,000 and the CTFA spent half a million dollars in 2005 opposing the safe cosmetics bill and other environmental health legislation in California.[4]

"The industry opposed this bill as though it were a peasant revolt rather than a right-to-know bill," said Andy Igrejas, environmental health director of the National Environmental Trust, which sponsored the bill along with the Breast Cancer Fund and Breast Cancer Action. Joining in support of the bill were Asian-American health groups, Catholic health care institutions and organized labor. With the bill in the high-profile hands of Governor Schwarzenegger, celebrities and teenage beauty queens stepped forward into the fray.

"Miss California Calls on Mr. Universe to Sign Cosmetics Safety Bill," announced the advisory for a press event featuring Miss California 2004 Veena Goel, who stood alongside Senator Migden and urged Governor Schwarzenegger to sign the bill. Melissa Gilbert, president of the Screen

Actors Guild, reminded the governor in a support letter that "actors are daily users of cosmetic products." Former Miss Teen World USA Sasha Hoffman joined five Marin County teenagers in an attempt to lobby the governor in person. Jessica Assaf described the experience of going to the state capitol in her essay "Lobbying":

> Walking up the stairs that tower over my head, I feel as unimportant as a speck of sand. I am overshadowed by the fear that I will not be heard, but as I enter the building, I do not look back. Holding a large white sign at my side, I place my bag on the table to be checked by the security guard. I can feel everyone's eyes target me and I imagine their judgments: Oh, just another stupid protester walking into the Capitol to fight for another stupid cause. Although my doubts begin to catch up to me as I remember I am only a 15-year-old lobbying against a billion-dollar industry, I continue walking with dignity. I pinch myself to get feeling back in my legs, which seem to be moving so quickly down the cold halls of the California Capitol. Is this really happening? ... I walk until I arrive at my destination: the office of Governor Arnold Schwarzenegger.[5]

The governor was out of town, the girls were told. Could they speak with someone else? As they waited, ignored for more than an hour, the girls began to feel hopeless as they stood outside the office holding their signs — "Teens should not have to choose between beauty and health" and "SB 484 must pass." Finally, the door cracked open and Schwarzenegger's deputy of cabinet affairs Kacy Hutchinson invited the teenagers inside. It was a critical moment. Opposition to the bill was so heated that the bill's supporters had not been able to make appointments to lobby the governor, according to Pete Price, the environmental lobbyist for the National Environmental Trust. But Price explained, "The girls had gained credibility by coming back again and again. To actually have kids on a school day standing outside his chambers, that's a story. The girls got access when nobody else did." The teens were given a chance to state their case, as Jessica Assaf explained to me later: "We were sitting in one of the big boardrooms and we just had five minutes to tell Kacy why this bill had to pass. It was the most amazing experience. You had to think on the spot, why is this important to me? So I just spoke from the bottom of my heart telling her why this bill really needed to pass."

The famous Republican governor was in a tight spot. On the one side, Schwarzenegger faced the wealthy cosmetics lobby. But could he really afford to veto a bill backed by breast cancer activists, teens, beauty queens, Catholics, actors and women in general — especially since he had picked (and lost) messy fights with California teachers and nurses during his first rocky year in office? Surprising even some of his closest allies, Schwarzenegger signed the California Safe Cosmetics Act into law October 8, 2005. David Crane, the governor's economic advisor and one of the few Democrats on his staff, had advised the governor to sign the bill, but Crane said Schwarzenegger's decision was, "believe me, entirely him ... I can guarantee you, there was incredible opposition to it, even among the staff. It was all him. He cared about it."

Under the new legislation, which went into effect January 1, 2007, cosmetics companies must disclose to the state if their products contain ingredients linked to cancer or birth defects; the state can also demand health-related information about cosmetic ingredients from manufacturers, and regulate products to protect salon workers if a risk is determined — all of which are good first steps toward safer cosmetics, but hardly revolutionary. "It's a lot of drama for a bill that seems rather modest, since it wouldn't ban any ingredients or require new labeling. It's about disclosure, period," as Marjie Lundstrom noted in her *Sacramento Bee* column.[6] Still it was, to date, the strongest law in the US regulating cosmetics. The environmental lobbyist Pete Price thinks the bill will drive some companies to quietly remove hazardous ingredients. "The fact that they're being required to publicly disclose, we hope that will cause many of them to reformulate their products because they don't want to deal with the grief," he said.

In the end, one of the more significant outcomes of the bill may be the impact it had on the girls who went to the California state capitol and learned that their opinion matters. "The girls really felt like they got that bill passed. For them to see they had the power and ability to do that, it was life changing for every one of us," said Judi Shils. "I had no idea about politics," Jessica Assaf told me. "I've always heard until you're 18 you have no rights, you can't vote, you have no influence on the government … But I do have a voice, I realize, and now I just want to keep on sharing it because I feel this is really important."

## Undercover, Part II

As the lobby drama played out in California one month before Schwarzenegger signed the bill, Susan Roll from the Massachusetts Breast Cancer Coalition was dusting off her Joyful business cards and heading back to New York City for Health and Beauty America 2005. In the year since her last undercover visit to this major industry conference, the Campaign for Safe Cosmetics had celebrated some key victories — top manufacturers had removed one of the worst ingredients from nail polish and the California legislature had passed a precedent-setting law. But these were small steps in the scheme of things. The Campaign for Safe Cosmetics decided to make that point with another full-page ad in *USA Today*. "Don't worry, I'm 11% tested," said the headline over a man who gazed pleadingly at a skeptical-looking woman. "Don't trust these odds? Then you should know: only 11% of the 10,500 chemicals *in your cosmetics* have been screened for safety." [7]

Susan again brought copies of the *USA Today* and placed them in strategic locations throughout the Jacob Javitz Conference Center, and she again headed to the panel on regulatory issues hosted by the Cosmetic, Toiletry, and Fragrance Association (CTFA). This time she noticed a different tone in the room. "It was much more complacent," Susan described, "more of a sense that the advocates were starting to be heard." [8]

The meeting kicked off with an inspiring speech by Pamela Bailey, the new president and CEO of the CTFA. Bailey spoke about her pride in the cosmetics industry and everything the industry had done for the health and well-being of women. "Beauty, health and safety of our customers is our number one priority every day," Bailey said. But Bailey observed that the industry was currently challenged by "increasing rumors and misinformation" about its products. It was CTFA's job to make accurate information available to consumers, she said.

Bailey asked Thomas J. Donegan, Jr., the CTFA vice president of legal and general counsel, to please speak to the "urban legend" that cosmetics aren't regulated. "At the end of the day, FDA has the same authority over cosmetics as it has over food and drugs," Donegan said. Bailey emphasized that there are stiff penalties and strict regulations for the cosmetics industry. This was indeed a different room from the year prior, when then-CTFA president Edward Kavanaugh began the meeting with the observation that "We are the most unregulated industry under the auspices of the FDA."

Next to speak at the meeting was Gerald McEwan, vice president of science at CTFA. He further emphasized all the FDA does to regulate cosmetics and explained that CTFA makes recommendations to the FDA every year about what the agency should focus on. The number one priority this year was responding to the petition filed by the Environmental Working Group, asking the FDA to recall cosmetics that violated the recommendations of the industry safety panel. The FDA was going to take its time responding to the petition, McEwan explained. They knew it was important and they would have to be careful.

The industry's biggest worry was, again, California. Lobbyist Mike Thompson talked about the difficult past 18 months and warned that this was just the beginning. The California Safe Cosmetics Act had passed through the legislature, Thompson reported, but they were optimistic the bill would be vetoed by Governor Schwarzenegger. "The next ten days will be a deciding point for this industry," he said. The best tactic for defeat was to show how the bill would hurt business in California. (The California legislature is "dysfunctional," Thompson said, which is why the opposition is able to make headway there. He later explained that although there were efforts in other states to regulate cosmetics, CTFA was mostly just watching California because "the legislatures of other states function better and we are stronger everywhere else.")

Someone in the audience wanted to know more about who was pushing for the California bill. Thompson replied, "Just look at the ad they took out in the newspaper; this is not a bunch of kids working out of a garage. They are well funded and can hire PR firms to do this kind of work." Susan has a vivid recollection of what happened next. Beauty consultant Rebecca Gadbury stood up from the audience and explained that the opponents weren't typical environmentalists. "This is the Breast Cancer Fund and that group in Marin where they have high rates of breast cancer. This is totally personal," Gadbury said. "The politicians are not voting on facts. They are voting because their mother died of breast cancer." A hush fell over the room, Susan recalled. "It was like there was this sudden understanding that these aren't just hippie liberals, these are people who are sick. This is mainstream America. Maybe we need to pay attention. There was a sense of confusion in the room, like people were wondering if they really did have the science to back up what they were saying."

## Miss Treatment USA

Some companies have a funny definition of the word "natural." OPI Natural Nail Strengthener, for example, had one of the highest toxicity ratings in the 2005 *Skin Deep* database — 11 different ingredients that raise health concerns, including the "toxic trio" of nail polish chemicals: toluene, formaldehyde and dibutyl phthalate.[9] You may not immediately place the name OPI, but call it "that nail salon brand" and most women nod their heads in recognition. With racy names like "Aphrodite's Nightie" and "I'm Not Really a Waitress," OPI nail products line the shelves of nail salons in 70 countries. The Los Angeles–based company is the largest manufacturer of nail polish and nail treatment products worldwide. This put OPI at the top of the list of toxic offenders. Day in and day out, women who work in nail salons — often women of color who are of childbearing age — were being exposed to hazardous chemicals that were a risk to developing fetuses. As the labor-union saying goes, when you're pregnant, every day is take your kid to work day.

OPI had already reformulated its products for the European market, removing dibutyl phthalate (DBP) to comply with the EU Cosmetics

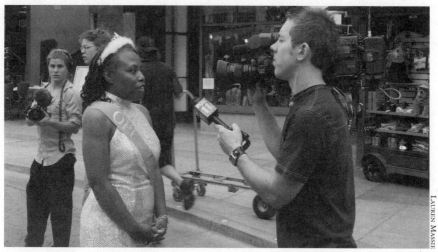

*Felecia Eaves, an organizer with Women's Voices for the Earth, talks to reporters, dressed as "Miss Treatment."*

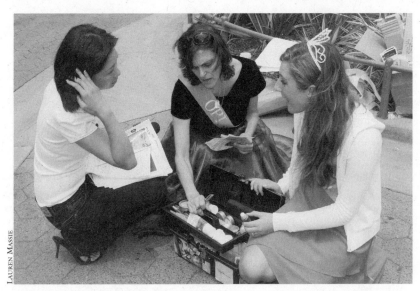

LAUREN MASSIE

*Judi Shils (middle) and Jessica Assaf (right) show a reporter the makeup kit of safer products at the Santa Monica Promenade "Miss Treatment" action.*

Directive. But the company was refusing to take the chemical out of US products. In February 2006, members of the Campaign for Safe Cosmetics had a phone meeting with Eric Schwartz, chief operating officer of OPI, to discuss the matter. Schwartz was "cordial," according to Felicia Eaves, an organizer with Women's Voices for the Earth who participated in the meeting.[10] "They've always been cordial. But the basic tone was that we have expert scientists and our scientists have said the levels of chemicals we have in our products do not pose a hazard. So we're not going to take it out. They felt DBP enhanced their product in terms of the longevity of the product," Felicia said. "We asked if the products they sold in Europe were inferior and they outright said yes, they thought it was an inferior product."

The campaign requested an in-person meeting, and in March 2006, Felicia, Charlotte Brody, Bryony Schwan and Janet Nudelman flew down to LA to meet with Schwartz.[11] Charlotte gave a presentation about the science of DBP. The OPI executives stood firm. They were not going to remove DBP from their products, they said, although they agreed to revisit the issue later in the year because the state of California was planning to list DBP as a known reproductive toxicant under the state's Proposition

65 law, which meant products containing the chemical above a "safe" exposure level might have to carry a warning notice. "Our feeling was that they were not going to do it until they were absolutely forced to do it," Felicia said. "So we decided to target them, in the sense of getting the public to put pressure on them to take the chemicals out."

The Campaign for Safe Cosmetics wrote up fact sheets about OPI products and hand delivered them to salons in a dozen cities. A full-page ad featuring a beauty queen named "Miss Treatment" ran in the *LA Weekly*, the hometown paper of OPI headquarters, and *Variety* magazine. "US Women awarded with some of the world's most toxic nail products!" said the caption beneath the happily waving beauty queen.[12] The ad promoted

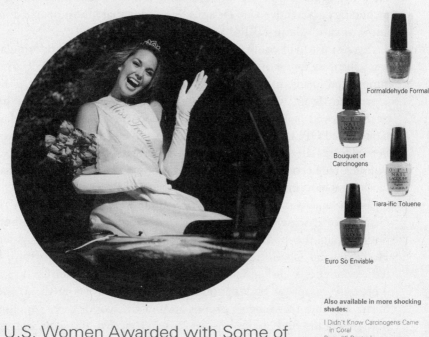

*Miss Treatment USA illustrated the fact that companies were selling safer nail products in Europe. A version of this ad ran in* Variety *and the* LA Weekly.

"OPI's Miss Treatment USA Series, with stunningly low American health standards." Spoofing the brand's quirky names, the ad suggested new names such as "Formaldehyde Formal" and "I Didn't Know Carcinogens Came in Coral." Miss Treatment also hit the road in the spring with a street theater action on the Santa Monica Promenade featuring a dozen women and teens dressed as beauty queens in hot pink sashes that read "OPI Miss Treatment." The action was covered on Fox TV and the Asian TV network, and hundreds of letters were sent to the company.[13]

The company stuck to its guns. In a story published in July 2006 in the *Pittsburgh Post-Gazette,* LaMont Jones reported, "OPI has no plans to remove DBP from polishes sold in the United States, saying that the level is so low that it poses no health risk."[14] Douglas Schoon, a nail product formulator, told Jones that the real victim in the story was dibutyl phthalate. "This is all just a political snafu that this poor ingredient has been caught in," said Schoon, vice president of science and technology at Creative Nail Designs. He added that "most people don't know or care" about DBP.

By August, nail companies that had not committed to reformulate were showing signs of caring. Leading drugstore brand Sally Hansen announced plans to reformulate all its products to remove DBP, formaldehyde and toluene. Orly International announced that DBP had been removed from its products too. When *LA Times* reporter Marla Cone called OPI to ask about their stance on the issue, the company told her they had already started taking DBP out of their products. "Nail Polishes to Become a Little Safer," reported the Campaign for Safe Cosmetics in a press release dated August 30, 2006.[15]

From that warm day in October 2000 when scientists from the Centers for Disease Control first reported finding high levels of dibutyl phthalate in the bodies of American women — from the day Jane Houlihan and Charlotte Brody first started tracking the labyrinth of toxic cosmetics — it had taken nearly six years, a European Union law, a pressure campaign by a national coalition of activists in the United States with ties to women's groups around the world, three expensive newspaper ads and major media coverage across the US; but the Campaign for Safe Cosmetics could claim a victory. Dibutyl phthalate — the potent reproductive toxicant or the "poor ingredient caught in a political snafu," depending on your perspective — was finally banished from nearly every major nail polish brand in the United States.

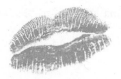

# 8

# Tricks of the Trade

Trade association: an association of people or companies
in a particular business or trade, organized to promote
their common interests.

— *Random House Unabridged Dictionary*, 2006

On her second day on the job, Pamela Bailey, the new president of
the Cosmetic, Toiletry, and Fragrance Association (CTFA), got a
call from Dan Brestle, president of the Estée Lauder Companies, Inc. "I
thought, when I was told he was on the phone, how nice, he's calling
to welcome me," Pamela told the crowd assembled in Boca Raton,
Florida for the 2006 CTFA annual meeting. "Which he did, for about
two sentences. And then he said, 'But that's not why I called. I'm *really
worried* about California.' Well, let me tell you, in only two days on the
job, I had reached the same conclusion. In a few short days, this industry's environment had dramatically changed." [1]

The dramatic change, the introduction of the California Safe Cosmetics
Act, occurred just a few days before Bailey took the helm of the US cosmetics industry's trade association. "We had to get to work fast to keep up with
this new landscape. We had our work cut out for us. We needed a strategic plan. We needed a road map." Bailey set four immediate priorities:

1. Prevent the California legislation. "Failure to prevent such legislation, we knew, would increase your costs, damage the industry's credibility and inhibit the very innovations that benefit consumers."

2. Enhance the industry's self-regulatory program to increase credibility.

3. Establish the trade association as the visible spokesperson for the industry.

4. Globally harmonize regulations and take "unified industry positions around the world on ingredients."

By March 2006, CTFA had already made good progress. Though they were unable to prevent the California Safe Cosmetics Act, the industry "mobilized unprecedented communications, grassroots and policy efforts," according to Pamela Bailey, and "together we achieved a bill in California that was much improved from the original proposal."

CTFA had also been on a hiring spree: new lobbyists on staff included John Herson, former majority leader of the Maryland General Assembly, and Elvis Oxley, son of US Congressman Mike Oxley (R–Ohio) and former director of the Ripon Society, a Republican lobby group. Oxley would join the DC lobby effort, freeing up lobbyist Mike Thompson to "fight 24-7 in California." A new stepped-up communications plan would be spearheaded by Kathleen Dezio, who was "fresh from similar challenges in the beverage industry."[2] The new staffers rounded out a roster at the trade association that illustrates the thin line between US government and industry. CTFA top staff includes John Bailey, who spent 30 years at FDA's Office of Cosmetics and Colors, and Alan Anderson, a 22-year FDA veteran now in charge of the industry's self-regulatory body, the Cosmetic Ingredient Review panel. All their government experience would no doubt come in handy as the cosmetics industry faced increasing regulatory challenges over toxic ingredients. However, as Pamela Bailey noted in her speech, "The new reality, unfortunately, when you look at the federal budget, is that there will be no federal funding available to FDA — either this year or in the foreseeable future — to focus on cosmetics." Pause. "That's *because* cosmetics and personal care products are the very safest products that FDA regulates. But we also know that industry needs FDA as the tough cop on the beat to protect us, and to reassure consumers."

## Spin Cycle

It's an interesting turn of phrase, "industry needs FDA as the tough cop on the beat to protect us." Isn't the tough cop on the beat supposed to protect us, the American public? Unfortunately, the FDA has little authority and few resources to oversee cosmetics safety. However, the agency does fulfill the role of reassuring consumers, according to a focus group commissioned by the cosmetics industry and conducted by Republican messaging guru Frank Luntz. Best known for his polling to develop the language for the 1994 Republican "Contract with America" and his work to reframe the estate tax as the "death tax," Frank Luntz conducted focus groups for both the cosmetics and chemical industries in 2006, using his famous "dial technology" to gauge the emotional reactions of focus group participants.

A "scare meter" is what Lexie Schultz called it.[3] For three hours, Lexie sat in a focus group conducted by Luntz in Washington DC in the spring of 2006. "Turn the dial to 100 if this scares the crap out of you, and zero doesn't worry you at all," the moderator told Lexie and the 27 other focus group participants. They were instructed to turn their dials to the left if they felt negatively and to the right if they felt positively about what they were hearing in a series of video clips. The first clip featured the Environmental Working Group raising concerns about phthalates in cosmetics. Most of the focus group participants had not heard of phthalates.

Every other video was from the cosmetics industry's point of view. The cosmetics industry tested out different spokespeople and messages, including some over-the-top descriptions of environmental groups that didn't play too well with the focus groups. "Chemical terrorist groups are trying to frighten you" by claiming that cosmetics are not safe, said one unidentified person in a video clip. "Extremist groups are cherry picking chemicals to make it seem like there's a problem," said another. "The more they used those extreme terms, the more they were seen as defensive," Lexie explained. Another theme, personal choice, also didn't fly with the focus group. In response to an argument that adults should be allowed to make their own decisions about cosmetic products as they do about alcohol and tobacco, participants asked, "Didn't the tobacco industry lie to us for years?" Other industry lines tested on the focus groups included:

- *People have been using these products for decades with no problems.*
- *We only get 150 consumer complaints a year about minor things like rashes.*

- *We list our ingredients so consumers have a choice.*
- *We've spent millions of dollars on scientific studies to ensure our products are safe.*

The last line went over well, according to Lexie. "The science message was the strongest in the room because people had the least independent knowledge of science."

The focus group participants also had clear preferences for which messengers they were likely to believe. Last on the list were obvious industry spokespeople. "They really hated the company spokesperson," Lexie said. They reacted most favorably to independent experts — a female epidemiologist went over especially well — and to government agencies. "People were willing to believe FDA," Lexie said. "The FDA comforted people." Comments from participants included "FDA is strong," and "Nothing would get through FDA if it wasn't safe." The participants reacted neutrally or favorably to environmental groups. Most said they would listen to what the groups had to say, but would also probably do their own research. The theme of research was probed throughout the session, as the moderator asked how people would do research and whom they would believe. Participants were asked to fill out worksheets describing a website with information about cosmetics ingredients to be launched in 2007.

Other themes tested on the focus group were along the lines of *Europe is weird* and *precaution is silly.* They are more hysterical in Europe than we are, the participants were told; Europe has decided some chemicals can't be in products, but the decisions were based on politics, not science, and European products are now less effective. The precautionary principle — the idea of basing decisions on the concept of "better safe than sorry" — *may seem like common sense, but it's not common sense.* Those messages met with some eye rolling in the room. The participants were skeptical of obvious company lines, Lexie confirmed. But many also acknowledged positive feelings about personal care products. "These products make my life simpler and more comfortable," said one participant. "I feel favorably because I depend on them a lot," said another. "They are marketing driven and generate a sense of unnecessary need," commented one participant, while another said: "We're not dropping dead; my face isn't rotting off. I'd rather roll the dice than walk around with my armpits stinking."

At the end of the day, the whole focus group exercise had a bit of a backfire element to it, in Lexie's view. "After three hours of using their messages, they asked how many people in the room were more concerned now [about cosmetics safety] than when they arrived. Half the people raised their hands."

## Cop on the Beat

> The FDA routinely conducts studies and tests to ensure the safety of all cosmetic products ... FDA's legal authority over cosmetics is comparable with its authority over other FDA-regulated products, such as foods, nonprescription drugs, and nonprescription medical devices.

Well, not really. These claims were posted on the CTFA website as of January 2007.[4] In reality, cosmetics are the least regulated products at the FDA. The agency does not routinely safety test cosmetic products; and unlike drugs, the agency doesn't require manufacturers to demonstrate cosmetic products are safe. CTFA has fought long and hard to keep it that way. In the 1970s, for example, CTFA "found itself in a decade-long struggle to convince regulatory agencies and consumer groups that the industry's commitment to product safety and self-regulation precluded the need to introduce new legislation," according to the association's website.[5]

A major threat came in 1973 when US Senator Thomas Eagleton (D-Missouri) proposed sweeping changes to federal oversight of the cosmetics industry. The Eagleton Bill would have mandated FDA pre-market clearance of cosmetics and required manufacturers to perform thorough toxicological tests before they could sell their products to consumers. The bill would cause "a serious misallocation of the nation's scientific resources," CTFA chairman Dick Edmondson told the US Senate. Unfortunately for CTFA, the FDA was at that time considering a petition to require labeling of cosmetic products. "Not wanting to appear to oppose both the consumer's right to know with regard to ingredient labeling and the perceived pro-consumer provisions of the Eagleton bill, CTFA decided to work with FDA to develop a regulation on ingredient labeling both sides could agree on," according to the CTFA website. Partial product labeling for cosmetics (with a huge loophole exempting fragrance ingredients) was thus achieved. And in lieu of the standardized toxicological testing proposed by the Eagleton Bill, the industry proposed the self-monitoring Cosmetic Ingredient Review panel, which in 30 years has reviewed just a fraction of cosmetic ingredients and found the vast majority to be "safe as used." Thomas Eagleton knew that was not going to be good enough. "Self-regulation of any kind is a myth," the former senator said. "FDA knew we were right, but finally concluded that they were already overwhelmed in other regulations."[6]

## The Trade Association Way

> Doubt is our product since it is the best means of competing with the "body of fact" that exists in the mind of the general public.
>
> — *1969 memo, written by an executive at*
> *Brown & Williamson tobacco company*[7]

For half a century, the tobacco industry muddied the link between smoking and cancer by funding skeptics, researching alternative explanations for lung cancer and mounting public relations campaigns to "manufacture doubt" about science.

"There's a saying in the PR business that for every PhD there's an equal and opposite PhD. And if there's not one then you can create one through funding. And if you put a lot of money into manufacturing ignorance, it can actually work," said Robert Proctor, history professor at Stanford University. "We saw this in tobacco, and we've seen it in polluting industries and global warming. There are lots of people out there who'd rather have you not know what's really going on."[8]

The chemical industry, for instance: two notorious examples of "lying to us for years" are documented in the 2002 book *Deceit and Denial: The Deadly Politics of Industrial Pollution*, by historians Gerald Markowitz and David Rosner.[9] The book is based on internal industry documents, including company memos and minutes from trade association meetings. It reveals how the Lead Industries Association, when faced with mounting scientific evidence that lead-based paint was harming children, launched an extensive marketing campaign to promote the use of lead paint in homes and hospitals — even targeting children with the ads. The campaign featured the cute little "Dutch Boy," happily painting away.[10]

*Deceit and Denial* also reveals how the chemical industry orchestrated an international cover-up to hide evidence that vinyl chloride monomer, the building block of vinyl plastic, was causing catastrophic injuries in plant workers.[11] A known carcinogen, vinyl chloride monomer was also used in propellant hair sprays at the time — and quietly removed with no warnings to women who had been routinely spraying themselves with a highly dangerous chemical.[12] The vinyl cover-up was the subject of a two-hour PBS documentary by Bill Moyers that aired in 2001, "Trade Secrets." At the end of the film, the chemical industry representative insisted that what happened 40 years ago is no reflection on the industry today.[13] Yet in 2005, the Environmental Protection Agency fined Du Pont $16.5 million for covering up two decades' worth of company studies about the health risks of a Teflon chemical that is ubiquitous in drinking water supplies and people's bodies.[14] Recent Du Pont ads in *Good Housekeeping* magazine feature a smiling young woman in a white lab coat with the caption, "As a scientist, I make Teflon. As a mother I use it."[15]

The line between the cosmetics industry and chemical industry is thin. Before taking the cosmetic industry's top job, Pamela Bailey spent six years as head of AdvaMed, the medical device manufacturers trade association. During that time, the group lobbied to keep vinyl medical devices — a major source of phthalate exposure to sick patients — unregulated and unlabelled. AdvaMed and the CTFA use the same "phthalates are safe" talking points as the Phthalates Ester Panel and the Vinyl Institute, trade associations that share offices with the chemical industry trade group, the American Chemistry Council. ACC recently launched a $35 million ad campaign called "chemicals are essential". The flagship ad, running in all the major opinion leader magazines, features a sick baby in an incubator full of plastic tubes.[16]

## Game Plan

The cosmetics industry has a long history of evading government oversight by proposing self-regulation schemes. In the new landscape of rising public concern about toxic chemicals, the trade association was reaching into a familiar bag of tricks. Their plan was announced at the 2006 CTFA meeting in Boca Raton:

1. Step up the industry's voluntary safety program with a new voluntary pledge, to be signed by all CTFA members, called the "Consumer Commitment Code."

2. Enhance the industry's self-policing Cosmetic Ingredient Review program.

3. Launch a new consumer-friendly website with scientific information about cosmetic ingredients.

The industry's counter move to the Compact for Safe Cosmetics and the *Skin Deep* website would be launched in 2007. Pamela Bailey summed up the goals of the new campaign. With the new high-power lobby team "we're going to take the facts to the policy-makers in other states about the strong FDA regulatory standards and the reliable science that we all know is behind each of your products." With the new website and stepped-up communications plan "we will be the source of information for our consumers, and it will be factual, science-based information, not misstatements and half-truths."

Despite the challenges that lay ahead, Bailey reassured the industry that they were entering the new era from a position of strength. And they could count on CTFA to protect their interests. "Our operating plan has a very clear purpose: it is to enable you to drive your own company's agenda, and to control your own destiny and to strengthen your own deep connection to your consumers."

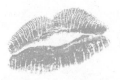

# 9

# *Unmasked*

Health and Beauty America 2006 — I was finally going to get a close-up look at the inner philosophies of the beauty industry. This year it was my turn to go undercover to the industry's largest gathering to listen in on the trade association's lobbying plans. Unlike Susan Roll, I didn't make up fake business cards for a company named Joyful; however, in order to avoid being turned away in case someone recognized my name, I used my mother's credit card for the $595 registration fee. The trade association's regulatory panel was a full-day event this year — the First Annual HBA Regulatory Summit.

"A history-making proactive initiative," was the way moderator Meyer Rosen explained the day. "We are really out to make a difference in this regulatory arena."[1] I leafed through the six-inch-thick binder in front of me containing the 17 PowerPoint presentations to come. I could already tell the cosmetics industry was more organized about running a meeting than the typical environmental group. But I was already disappointed. I expected flash and sizzle — slick video, neon signs, goodie bags, something. This was, after all, the cosmetics industry. Instead, here we were in a beige basement room under fluorescent lights with nothing to look at but the dour faces of mostly bald men on the panel.

The first speaker, Bruce Ames, PhD, professor of the graduate school of biochemistry and molecular biology at the University of California, set the philosophical framework for the day in a presentation entitled "Putting Cancer Risks in Perspective."

## Choose Your Poison

Dr. Ames zipped through a series of complicated slides about cellular cytoplasm and mitochondrial matrix and then got straight to the point: we're living longer, there's no need to worry about parts per billion of pesticides, the real problem is poor diets and micronutrient deficiencies (and by the way he has a company that sells multivitamins and mineral pills). He is most concerned about Vitamin D deficiencies.

According to Dr. Ames' slide presentation:

### The Causes of Cancer

30% smoking

35% unbalanced diets: too many calories, obesity, too
    little fiber/micronutrients

20% chronic infections: mostly in poor countries

20% hormones: breast, endometrial, etc. [no mention
    of hormone-disrupting chemicals]

2% occupation

<1% pollution: mostly heavy air pollution

The real problem is that people are eating a "horrible diet of refined everything." Dr. Ames is helping people to "see through all this confusion of worrying about parts per billions of pesticides and not the important things," like for example, "people with rickets." Doctors hadn't seen cases of rickets for 50 years, but now because of Vitamin D deficiencies, 60 cases of rickets were diagnosed in children's hospitals last year. Folic acid deficiency can give you cancer, and iron deficiencies can cause brain damage. "The poor are eating these horrible diets, and I think they're making their kids stupid." Biotin deficiency, zinc deficiency, magnesium deficiency are all problems. "Anytime you are deficient in micronutrients throughout life you're taking it out of DNA and aging faster and getting cancer."

Dr. Ames explained that black people are not getting enough sun in the US. All African Americans have Vitamin D deficiency and they consequently have higher rates of cancer. Slathering on sunscreen is not such a good idea. We've gone too far with sunscreen because we're not

getting enough Vitamin D. This is a "coming public health disaster in the US." Everyone should
get a half hour of sunshine a day.

"People say the cancer rates are increasing,
that's all nonsense." To illustrate the point, he
showed several slides of declining cancer deaths.[2]
Natural and synthetic substances have the same
cancer "hit rates." A number of natural chemicals
in coffee and volatile chemicals in tomatoes are
carcinogens. "The idea that science and technology are doing us in and if only we'd go back to
nature we'd be fine — people forget that cars are
safer than horses," Dr. Ames said. Ninety-nine
percent of the scare stories in the paper about toxic
chemicals are wrong. "Newspapers like scare stories, intellectuals don't like capitalism and there's
nothing to it."

## Who Is Behind the Hype?

Next up was Rebecca James Gadbury, the president of YG Laboratories, who offered interesting
explanations about what she called the "Toxic
Ingredients Movement." Gadbury was raised on
Rachel Carson and started out being a Mary Kay
girl when she was 10. When it comes to the Toxic
Ingredients Movement, she is not an apologist
but an explainer.

Gadbury showed a slide with newspaper headlines generated by the Campaign for Safe Cosmetics
and asked: Who is behind the hype?

- The bored & the lonely with Internet
  connections
- Cosmetic companies profiling their unique-
  ness against their competition
- Non profit "Watch Dog" organizations who
  survive on donations of "motivated" donors
- Scientifically naïve journalists seeking "eyes"

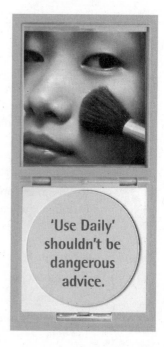

**'Use Daily' shouldn't be dangerous advice.**

**150 cosmetics companies agree: Beauty products don't need to be toxic.**

Every day, we use as many as 25 personal
care products on our bodies. Some of the
chemicals in these products are linked to
cancer, infertility and birth defects—and
most have never been evaluated for their
health effects.

More than 150 cosmetics companies are
leading the way in cleaning up their industry.
These companies have signed a pledge—
the Compact for Safe Cosmetics—to remove
hazardous ingredients. Now, all cosmetics
companies should sign the Compact and
prove that their concern for their customers
is more than just skin deep.

**Has your favorite brand pledged to make safe products?**

The Campaign for Safe Cosmetics
www.SafeCosmetics.org

Big Think

The nonprofit groups are "earning money by selling fear," Gadbury said. "Just like my uncle, the insurance salesman, they convince everybody they're going to die and then sell them insurance." (The theme was repeated throughout the day, with several speakers referring to environmental groups that are "in it for the money.")

What's driving the Toxics Ingredients Movement? The internet is the great leveler making everyone's opinion as valuable as everyone else's; industry no longer has a one-way conduit of information to consumers. Also there are improvements in our ability to understand how cosmetic ingredients are affecting the body and our environment, plus we live in a chemophobic society.

Gadbury presented chemical facts to share with non-chemists:

- Everything in the world is made of chemicals (except light and electricity).
- There is no such thing as a "chemical-free cosmetic."
- All natural cosmetics are made of chemicals.
- Here is the most important thing to remember: All cosmetic ingredients are CHEMICALS (another word for "ingredient" is "chemical").

To be fair, these environmental organizations are concerned about carcinogenic, mutagenic and fetal toxicants; aggregate exposure to chemicals; chemical mixtures; and worker exposures to high levels of suspect chemicals. "Many ingredients are not tested for this." The groups want products reformulated to eliminate known or probable carcinogens, mutagens and fetal toxicants regardless of exposure levels in one product. "That's impossible but that is what they want." They're "concerned by presence, not by parts per billion/million."

She warned the industry "It is no longer enough to say 'cosmetics are inherently safe' … Every time I hear someone say 'cosmetics are safe' I want to strangle them because there's no proof. The fact that we've used them for years and can't track bad things to them does not mean they are inherently safe … At this point in the industry's technology, no one can make a product 100% safe." As one of the few self-regulating industries left, we must take on the responsibility of regulating ourselves. If we regulate ourselves and we rise to the occasion, we will all benefit monetarily and as well be able to look ourselves in the mirror in the morning. She recommended that everyone develop a Safe Ingredient Strategy:

- Remove all ingredients recognized by California as carcinogens or fetal toxicants in scientifically valid studies regardless of percentage or length of exposure.
- Ask ingredient vendors to provide available ingredient data regarding carcinogenicity, mutagenicity and fetal toxicity.
- Investigate and adopt a "green chemistry" policy to whatever degree that is possible.
- Adhere to a product safety policy.

## European Trendsetters

In the final presentation of the morning, on "Emerging Global Regulatory Trends," Ken Rivlin from the Allen and Overy law firm explained that although the US used to be a worldwide leader in environmental policy, the EU is now at the forefront of environmental policy-making. Europe doesn't look at cost/benefit analysis but instead uses the "do no harm" precautionary principle: "If it's going to cause a problem, don't do it." The US approach, in contrast, is: "If we want to do it, we're going to do it, unless there's a real good reason why we shouldn't."

According to Rivlin, Europe is different because of

- Different consumer views: "In Europe the citizenry feels differently about the environment than we do; it's a more green culture."
- Different political system — proportional representation (versus the US "winner take all" system).
- Different law-making processes.

The difference in approach can be seen in the way the two continents regulate cosmetics: The EU law has negative ingredient lists (of banned chemicals) and specific testing and data requirements for cosmetic ingredients. In contrast the US has few ingredient restrictions and the manufacturers are responsible for testing. "The EU model is taking over the world." Many countries have reproduced aspects of the EU Cosmetics Directive: approximately 50 countries have adopted the EU cosmetic definition; about 30 countries have adopted the EU "negative ingredient" lists. Other EU regulatory approaches were also being globally adopted, such as a directive that bans highly toxic substances from electronic equipment. China, Japan, South Korea and California were adopting similar legislation. "We see this trend of the EU being a frontrunner."

On the horizon in Europe, the major development is the new chemicals legislation called REACH — for "Registration, Evaluation and Authorization of Chemicals." The REACH legislation requires the chemical industry to provide safety data for thousands of high-volume chemicals and substitute the most hazardous chemicals. In Rivlin's opinion, REACH would not have a major impact on the cosmetics industry.[3] On the horizon in the United States: the trade association's new consumer commitment initiatives and "a new global communications infrastructure for harmonizing global regulations." Another important global trend is the increased focus on green marketing, organic products and environmental stewardship. Rivlin concluded: "It's not all doom and gloom. Take the challenges and turn them into opportunities."

## The Organic Element

At lunchtime, I avoided mingling with the crowd. With all the icy stares from the podium directed at my note-taking, I was nervous that I'd get tossed out or worse. So I headed upstairs for a quick trip around the trade show floor. This was no thumping, buzzing, freebie product-pushing lovefest like California's Natural Products Expo. The Health and Beauty America crowd was more subdued, approaching disaffected, as they lingered fashionably behind glass counters. If one thing caught my attention, it was those counters: elaborate display cases featuring empty colored bottles twinkling like jewels under the spotlights. The place was a shrine to packaging obsessed with youth and sexual appeal. Everyone and everything at HBA, it seemed, invoked the anti-aging dream — wrinkle-free claims at every product booth, even wrinkle-free jokes mixed in with the morning presentations.

I found a booth for organic ingredients and asked the proprietor, "Do you get much interest in organics from the big companies?" He dropped into a trance-like sales pitch and told me that organic ingredients are proven to boost the natural anti-aging capabilities of the body. But the pitch didn't last long — he could tell I was not a buyer — so he shrugged and told me the big companies are interested in organics, all right, but they're mostly interested in the cheapest ingredients they can find. And if they become very interested in an organic ingredient, the result is a degraded ingredient, which is what happened with aloe vera.

I made a brief stop at the booth of the Cosmetic, Toiletry, and Fragrance Association. The man behind the counter was very friendly and wanted to talk. "Are you a member? You really should join up," he said, and handed me the benefits brochures. Membership dues are based on a sliding scale of $625 a year for the smallest companies up to $397,500 plus a percentage of sales for companies with more than $2 billion in cosmetics sales. I did a quick calculation on my way back down to the basement and figured that the trade association dues for just one member, Procter & Gamble, would exceed the entire annual budget of the Campaign for Safe Cosmetics.[4]

## The Big Safety Plan

Now it was time to hear the details about the trade association's new Consumer Commitment Code from John Bailey, former head of the FDA cosmetics office and current vice president of scientific affairs of the Cosmetic, Toiletry, and Fragrance Association. Bailey, said moderator Meyer Rosen, "has always been on our side, even when he worked with the FDA. He was always willing to give an inside voice." Previous speakers had joked about Bailey being "user friendly" to industry during his tenure at FDA. "If I'd known I was so user friendly I would have been a bit tougher," Bailey joked in return.

"Cosmetics are the safest products FDA regulates," Bailey said, "and that's why they are the least regulated. It is a terrific model for public-private partnerships." After many board meetings, CTFA had decided to launch a new safety initiative. Bailey explained how the plan would work, and how companies should demonstrate the safety of their products:

1. Consumer Commitment Code: All CTFA members would be required to sign the Code; however, Bailey stressed that compliance with the program is voluntary. Companies would agree to:

   • Inform the FDA of any serious and unexpected adverse experience from the use of the product in the US (hospitalization, disfigurement, etc.).

- Maintain a summary of information about product and ingredient safety. Bailey explained the criteria for documenting safety: if there is a Cosmetic Ingredient Review panel conclusion on an ingredient "stop there, you don't have to go any further." If there is no CIR conclusion, it would be sufficient to use "something in your file that talks about the safety of the ingredient of that product," such as a "statement from a supplier or your own risk assessment."

- Make the safety information available to the FDA upon request. Requests must be made in writing by an FDA district director. Bailey assured the companies that CTFA will "make sure these are legitimate requests and not just fishing expeditions." These will be "pretty rare events ... I don't think they're going to be lining up at the door ... [but] in talking to my former colleagues at FDA, they are aware of this and they are going to be knocking on some doors."

2. New industry website: The new CTFA website will enable consumers to search for cosmetic ingredients and get a message about safety. "We will craft that message in different ways," Bailey said, with information that will "tell both sides of the story" — the "more difficult to deal with" information would be "put in a context of products and safety."

3. Enhancements to the Cosmetic Ingredient Review panel: The CIR panel will "move faster through ingredients with transparency and enhance communications to make their website more user-friendly."

"This is just a continuation and looking at it in the current light and positioning for the future," Bailey concluded.

## Toxicity: A Moving Target

The next speaker provided a contrasting viewpoint to all the previous talk about cosmetics safety. Harold Zeliger, a toxicologist at Zeliger Chemical Environmental and Toxicological Services, conceded that many cosmetics contain toxic components. "If they weren't toxic we wouldn't be here," he said.

A partial list of toxic chemicals in cosmetics from Zeliger's paper includes:

- *Preservatives:* formaldehyde, quaternium-15, methyl and propyl paraben
- *Antioxidants:* butylatedhydroxyanisol (BHA), butylatedhydroxytoluene
- *Ointment bases:* lanolin alcohol, propylene glycol, polyethylene glycol
- *Emulsifying agents:* sodium lauryl sulfate, glyceryl stearate, cetyl alcohol

"We all know that some of these chemicals are toxic" and that mixtures present dangers that are not always predictable, Zeliger said. Weird things happen with chemical mixtures; there can be wildly high toxicities and people get sick in strange ways. "Mixtures seem to have a life of their own. One has to start thinking of a mixture as an entity in and of itself. It's not A plus B. It's C," Zeliger said. "This points out the need to retest whenever you change any formulation." When you change things, and you've all experienced this, you start getting phone calls: "I got a rash" or "my eyes are burning."

The FDA, Zeliger confirmed, has no testing requirements. The FDA "sort of suggests you may want to test but doesn't require it," nor does it define what tests are to be carried out. "This is incredible ... FDA will ultimately be forced to extend their regulations. But FDA is not equipped to regulate." The FDA has known since 1988 about the dangers of hydroquinone (the ingredient in skin lightening creams), that it absorbs into the skin and is a precursor to benzene, but is just now getting around to doing anything about it.

Zeliger recommended that the industry "present the FDA with a new set of tough standards for testing and labeling." A benefit of this can be seen in the pesticides law. "Once they get sign-off by EPA, it's a free ticket out of any litigation." It's basically a "government stamp of approval." You could do the same thing with cosmetics — get the FDA to sign off on labels. "Don't view changing regulations as a one-time exercise. This is a moving target. Every day we know more about the toxicity of chemicals than we did the day before."

## The Little Problem
"In order to keep out the fighting and screaming we carefully kept out consumer groups," moderator Meyer Rosen explained when he introduced

George Kimbrell, a lawyer with the International Center for Technology Assessment. But Kimbrell was invited due to the importance of the FDA petition he had filed for Friends of the Earth — the first legal action in the US that attempts to mitigate the human and environmental risks of nanotechnology. The very small particles of nanotechnology were a health concern because of their potential to penetrate quickly and deeply into the body.

The "gold rush" for nanotechnology patents continues, with more than 4,000 US patents issued to date, Kimbrell reported. More than $32 billion in nano-products were sold in 2005, twice the amount as in 2004. There are now more than 200 self-identified nano-products on US shelves, including paints, sporting goods, sunscreens, cosmetics, stain-resistant clothing, cell phones and digital cameras. The personal care industry is leading the way as the largest single category. Companies using nano-materials include Almay, Barney's NY, Chanel, Clinique, Estée Lauder, Johnson & Johnson, L'Oréal, Lancôme, Revlon and many others.

The FDA treats nano-material ingredients no differently than bulk material ingredients. The agency believes the existing battery of toxicity tests is adequate for most nanotechnology products. Particle size is not the issue, according to the agency. This view is out of step with the entire scientific community. Size matters at the nano-scale. Nano is best understood to mean "fundamentally different." Kimbrell feels strongly that the FDA must act quickly if the agency hopes to avoid past regulatory failures such as asbestos, DDT and PCBs.

More environmental health studies are urgently needed. Only 4% of the $9 billion dedicated to nanotechnology research in 2006 went to environmental and health research. "What we're left with are early studies that raise warning flags and no follow-up," Kimbrell said. "We need a real regulatory framework that protects public health and the environment."

## Questions of Value

During the day's closing question-and-answer period, consumer advocate Kimbrell got a chance at the mike and bravely pushed forth with the idea of strong government regulations: "We believe FDA should be in charge of regulations, not the industry. To those who say their products are safe when they come to market, I'd say that's great, but I'd rather not take your word for it. Let's see the data." Toxicologist Zeliger, the other person on the panel who seemed to favor strong regulations, advised: "Rigorously read the [scientific] literature — and it changes every day. Don't make believe [the studies] don't exist. Look at them seriously."

But differences in philosophy were clear. Moderator David Steinberg found the whole question about product safety very strange. "How many people put unsafe products on the market? How many people buy them?" Steinberg lectured the room about labeling products "parabens free" — "Our industry advertises that our products are not safe! We have to stop self-destructing!" The next topic — the "whitening trend in Asia" — highlighted the differences in the room. The FDA was threatening to ban hydroquinone, the highly toxic ingredient in skin lightening creams. What should the industry do? "If you want to continue skin lightening, someone has to produce data to show it's safe, otherwise it's going to go away as a category," said Rebecca Gadbury. Someone suggested the FDA threat could be handled with labeling, in the way that benzyl peroxide is still allowed in acne treatment with additional warnings. But Zeliger strongly disagreed: "I think it's *arrogant* to take a known benzene metabolite and sell it to the public."

They wanted to know, what did Dr. Ames think? Ames had to agree that "covering your skin with hydroquinone makes me a little nervous." But Dr. Ruud Overbeek felt that the hazard didn't matter. "The hazard could be significant," he reminded everyone, but what matters is how much exposure there is. "The risk and benefit have to be weighed," he said, as many heads nodded in the room.

## At the End of the Day

I was standing outside the Javitz Center waiting for a taxi when Bruce Ames walked up and tossed his plastic name tag in a trash can in front of me with a snap of the wrist, like he was glad to be done with the whole ordeal. He eyed me wearily for an instant then headed off into the New York night. That moment is my lasting regret. I should have stopped him and asked: What happened? How is it that the guy who invented the Ames Cancer Test[5] 30 years ago is on the industry conference circuit telling companies that pollution doesn't matter and they should keep using toxic ingredients? I wondered if Dr. Ames had reviewed the research showing that synthetic chemicals can interfere with the body's absorption of micronutrients.

Ames was just one of many mysteries from this long strange day. Weird, for instance, that there was so much open acknowledgment about the changing market landscape — about the global trend toward precautionary laws, the rapidly emerging scientific knowledge about chemical toxicity and the rising consumer demand for eco-friendly products. Yet the US cosmetic industry's big plan for the future is to operate just as it has in the past.

Ideology covered the day like a wet blanket. We're living longer, there's no need to worry about parts per billion of pesticides, so let's just keep doing business as usual. Corporations get to make the decisions in this country and nobody can tell us otherwise. The toxic chemicals we use are safe, and if the public doesn't believe it, we just need to do a better job of educating them about the "context of product safety" — i.e., the low levels of toxins in this one product are safe if used as directed, according to the incomplete information available in our risk assessments or supplier statements.

Yet there was also fresh air in that basement room: George Kimbrell arguing for the precautionary principle, Harold Zeliger encouraging proactive attention to the scientific literature. Rebecca Gadbury, in the context of describing the threat of the Toxic Ingredients Movement, advocated for safety programs that are strikingly similar to those proposed by the Campaign for Safe Cosmetics, or at least a step in the right direction: she encouraged companies to remove ingredients recognized as carcinogens or fetal toxicants regardless of the level of toxins in the product,[6] to require comprehensive toxicity information from chemical suppliers and to adopt green chemistry programs. Was anybody upstairs listening?

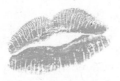

# 10

# A Healthier Foundation

"Cosmetics should be safe enough to eat," says Horst Rechelbacher, who founded Aveda, built it into the largest environmentally-friendly beauty salon in the US and then sold it to Estée Lauder Companies in 1997 for $300 million cash.[1] Now that his non-compete clause with Estée Lauder is up, Horst is getting back into the beauty business. "Should I sit back and become an activist and tell people what to do? No, you don't tell people what to do. You show them." So he started a new company to sell food-grade cosmetic products certified under the organic food standards. "If you wouldn't put it *in* your body, why would you put it *on* your body?" He sees no point in toxic ingredients.

The reason Horst waited so long to start a new product line was that he "didn't read the fine print in the contract" with Estée Lauder, which specified he had to quit and then wait five years before starting a competing business. He stayed on with Estée Lauder after the 1997 sale, hoping to use the big company's resources to reformulate products. "I thought it would be a great opportunity for me to clean up the cosmetics industry," Horst recalled. "Well it didn't work out that way ... How it was presented is that it's very costly to change products — hard to reformulate and relabel, and it's a big business interruption. It became a nonsense to me."

So Horst quit, waited the five years, and now the organic farmer from Wisconsin (with an apartment in Manhattan) will recreate the magic of a career that began more than 50 years ago in Austria. Horst got his first salon job at age 14, became a champion hair stylist winning prizes all over Europe and then opened his own salon in the 1960s. One day his mother, a herbalist, came to visit. "Horst, it smells terrible in here," she told him. At that moment something clicked for him, and everything changed. "If you're sitting on a mountain it's very difficult to see the mountain," he said, "if you smell it every day." He and his mom started experimenting with new formulations and making natural products. In the early 1970s, Horst "got turned on to Eastern philosophy" and went to India to study Ayurveda, a form of plant-based medicine that emphasizes prevention. That's where he came up with the name Aveda (Sanskrit for "all knowledge") and the idea to open a salon that sold products as free of toxins and petrochemicals as he could make them.

There were challenges. "There is no safe hair color, unfortunately," Horst explained. Some products starting to hit the market now are "50% safer but still toxic." He told the Aveda chemists he required a natural hair color and "they said they could do it, but they didn't." Now he's not inclined to trust the chemists, and he prefers to work with food scientists. His philosophy on product ingredients — "If it's not available in nature and in food, don't use it" — is extreme, even in the natural products industry. But he claims you can make just about everything from all-natural, food-grade ingredients except hair color, hair straighteners, hair permanents and sunscreen, none of which he plans to sell (except the sunscreen; he'll use zinc oxide).

Horst has seen surprisingly few innovations in cosmetics chemistry over the decades. Many companies are still using the "same old soap technologies" and toxic preservatives. In his view, the raw material providers hold the key to innovation in the cosmetics industry, and a big breakthrough needs to happen. "The chemical industry is also going to have to change. The world is changing," Horst said. He tried to tell this to his fellow business leaders during his keynote speech at a recent industry conference. More than 300 CEOs of all the major cosmetics companies were there. Horst pulled out a brochure from the Campaign for Safe Cosmetics and held it up in front of the room. "This is the customer. This is our intelligent customer," he told them. "And if we are not pleasing the customer, we are stupid. We are swimming against the river."

The activist groups, he said, "are called the cultural creatives, and it's one of the fastest growing consumer groups ... This new customer group is growing faster than your businesses right now."

Another customer nobody is paying attention to, he said, is Mother Earth. "If we slip from that, we become polluters. Healing Mother Nature is about healing ourselves. This is the business opportunity of the 21$^{st}$ century ... All we have to do is design new systems. That's new business." The CEOs gave him a standing ovation at the end of the speech, but the next day there was "a bit of backstabbing," he said, when other speakers rolled their eyes at "old Horst" and said "everything we do is safe, it's FDA approved, the same old stories."

But as he said, "you don't tell people what to do, you show them," and so his new venture will be "a little role model company so I can say, 'excuse me, if you need help, I'll give it to you'." Horst doesn't expect his new company, Intelligent Nutrients, to be the next Aveda empire. "Small is beautiful" is his new business philosophy, and his goal is to "help everybody to get there. It's possible and it's available. We can't be exactly what we've been in the past. It's time to reinvent the cosmetics industry."

## California Gold

Free organic soap, granola bars and a bottle of mint-infused water make their way into my canvas bag as I run the gauntlet of enthusiastic people lining the entrance to Natural Products Expo West. Inside on the floor of the Anaheim Convention Center, the business opportunity of the 21$^{st}$ century is on full display in all its mad glory: more than 3,000 booths offering tiny bottles of natural shampoo, morsels of organic food and other flashy tricks that make it hard to focus in any one direction. The place has the throng and pulse of an outdoor marketplace in Bangladesh, infused with the rush for California gold. This is an industry on the brink of the big time, and change is in the air. It's the era of the "new greening of America," as a *Newsweek* cover article[2] called it: eco-consciousness and natural products are in.

Though organic foods represent just 2% of total food and beverage sales in the US, the market is growing at a stunning 20% a year. Sales of natural cosmetic products are increasing faster than conventional product sales. Corporate America is paying attention. "By many accounts, the green business movement is taking off," wrote Michael S. Rosenwald in the *Washington Post,* "with the marketplace topping more than $228 billion in the United States and with such companies as Wal-Mart Stores Inc. getting into organic food and General Electric Co. plowing into renewable energy. Levi's is introducing organic cotton jeans. *Vanity Fair* recently published a green issue." [3]

Where the dollars flow, the largest corporations are sure to follow — and the inevitable question: how green is green going to be once Wall Street gets hold of it? The question hung heavy in the air, alongside the essential-oil fumes in the aisles of the world's largest trade show for natural and organic products. The Expo still attracts a diverse mix of small and owner-operated companies built on sweat equity and principles of social responsibility. But every year brings more stories of sell-outs to huge corporations: The Body Shop to L'Oréal, Aveda to Estée Lauder, Seeds of Change to M&M Mars, and the big news of 2006, Tom's of Maine to Colgate. "Nothing will change," said a rep at the Tom's booth in a near-defiant tone. But old-timers just shook their heads.

## We're All One or None

The first place to go for good stories is the booth with the magic soap. "You're sitting right here in one of the most shark-infested industries in America. There is quackery up the gazoo," said Ralph Bronner, son of legendary soap maker Dr. Bronner. "Any company reading your book could do what we've done tomorrow."

To Ralph that means "constructive capitalism," which he explained in his theatrical, run-on sentence kind of way: "Constructive capitalism is where you share the profit with the workers and the Earth from which you made it. You and I are brothers and sisters because of one eternal loving Father, and we should take care of each other and this planet. And that's why we have an orphanage we help in China, an orphanage in Haiti, freshwater wells in Ghana; we help the Chiapas Indians with schools; and David our president is taking on the federal government and fighting for legalized industrial hemp and organic standards — all to help the Earth."

If ever a company wore its values right on its sleeve, Dr. Bronner's Magic Soap is it. The company was founded by an eccentric German immigrant who spent his life on a modern-day Christian crusade. "He sold soap as a way to distribute the philosophy on the label," Ralph explained. "Jew or Gentile, everyone needs soap," Ralph recalls his father saying, "but the soap is just the messenger."

*We Are All One or None!*
*The whole world is our country, our fatherland, because all mankind is*
*born its Citizens!*
*Sow & you shall reap!*
*Work hard & you shall create!*
*Speak with Love, don't be afraid!*

The Moral ABCs, they call it, 3,000 words crammed onto a label of pure castile soap. The "soap with the funny label," as it is known. "They were the quotes my father loved from everyone who had a philosophy," explained Ralph Bronner, whose job it was to retype the label as the message evolved. "I was so sick of typing it that I told Dad, nobody is going to read this crap." But his father was determined to get the label exactly right. "Dad searched harder for God than anyone I know. Every night, he'd say I can't come to eat, I'm working on the Moral ABCs. What's more important, eating or uniting the Earth?"

Emmanuel Bronner, a self-proclaimed "doctor" from a line of master soap makers, started peddling soap from his tenement apartment in LA after escaping from a Chicago mental hospital where he received the shock treatments that he blamed for his 30 years of blindness. ("Hollywood could not make this up, it's real," Ralph explained.) In the 1960s, Dr. Bronner became an icon of the counterculture after hippies discovered they could use his 18-in-1 Pure-Castile Soap to wash clothes, degrease bikes and even brush teeth.

Today Dr. Bronner's soap company is worth $18 million and remains a family affair, despite at least 30 buyout offers. Company president David Bronner, Ralph's nephew, agreed to come on board only if he could clean up the product ingredients. "My father was not a saint," Ralph admitted. "I'll go to my grave not knowing how somebody sucked him into synthetic rose scent in a bottle of rose oil that said it was completely natural. David made our rose bar smell more like a rose than a rose. That's a symbol of David turning our business around." The products are now made entirely of organic food-grade ingredients, and the company gives 40-70% of profits to social and political causes. The highest paid employee makes no more than five times the lowest paid employee.

"We live the label," said Ralph. None of the above would be possible if they put the company on the stock market. "It sounds really nice, go public. Ask Ben and Jerry what it's like," Ralph commented. "Tom's is going to find this out by selling to Colgate. If you go for the numbers you're lost in the numbers, Mother Teresa. So the only way to do what you want, especially if you want to do something good for the Earth, is never sell out."

It's all so beautifully simple, according to Ralph Bronner. "To all of you who own a business or are a CEO, you can do what we're doing with two simple changes: create products so good that you don't have to spend fortunes marketing them, and share your profits and your salaries with the workers. It's almost too simple." Ralph tells these stories at schools and community events across the US, which is about the extent of the company's marketing program. At some point in each of his talks: "I grind to a halt and I say, 'take out your pencils and notebooks and I'll give you two words as a guide for life'. And I let them sit, because just like them you're thinking, what two words? And I don't think anyone guesses I'm going to say, 'Stay human.'"

## Beyond Organic

Mention the word "organic" at the Expo and get ready for the sparks to fly. The word has been hijacked! "My friend walked into Wal-Mart and saw polyester pajamas no doubt made by slaves in China that say 'Go Organic!' — that's the meaning of organic in America today," said Karen Ceisar, founder of Trillium Organics. Special interests pushing their own agendas have stolen the word "organic" and rendered it meaningless, according to Diana Kaye, founder of Terressentials. Diana more than believes cosmetics should be safe enough to eat; she'll show you — one time she dumped body oil on a muffin and ate it in front of reporters at a press conference. "Organic food standards are being dumbed down. The public has no idea what's going on," Diana said. But at least there are standards for organic food; in personal care products, "it's a total free-for-all."

As of spring 2007, there are no standards for organic personal care products in the US. The word "organic" — like the words "pure," "natural" and "gentle" — can be used as marketing claims on any personal care product, with no guidelines. For years, the organic purists have argued with the not-so-purists about creating an industry standard for organic personal care products. The ideal standards would "give the consumer what the consumer thinks they're paying for, and at the same time support family farmers by encouraging more businesses to source organic," explained Craig Minnowa, an environmental scientist with the Organic Consumers Association. Negotiations among interested parties have been ongoing, and a volunteer task force is close to recommending guidelines for a new organic seal for personal care products, which will likely allow for the use of some synthetic chemicals that meet specific criteria.[4]

Europe is, again, ahead of the game with standards for natural personal care products. One of the most prominent is BDIH, a German private-sector label for "Certified Natural Products." [5] The standard requires natural ingredients with a limited list of allowable synthetics; it rejects synthetic fragrances, dyes and petroleum products, as well as the commonly used preservative parabens. "If you don't get BDIH, don't even think about going to market in Europe" with a natural product, said Jennifer Barckley, public relations manager of Weleda North America. The Swiss-based company is the largest user of organic rose oil in the world, and the company meets its large demand for organic ingredients through fair-trade projects with farmers in several countries. "Originally we started working with 120 farmers who were growing roses conventionally, and we helped buy the equipment and helped to teach them the ways of organic agriculture," Jennifer said. "Now they are producing the rose petals that we need for all of our products. So we benefit, they benefit and it's just a great partnership." In the US, the word organic "is abused a lot," Jennifer observed. "I think that the US is a little bit behind and I think it's just a matter a time ... It's important to have standards."

## The Heart of the Matter

Bruce Akers pulled little glass vials out of a cardboard box and offered to make me some perfume. Spearmint and ylang ylang mix well together, he said, minty but sweet. Depending on his mood, he might add cedar wood to lemongrass. But his secret favorite, don't tell anyone, is vetiver, lavender and black pepper. As a chemist, Bruce Akers is naturally fond of chemicals. As a formulator of natural products, he's supportive of the people who make and buy such products. But Bruce has a cynical sense about him that applies to all of the above. He says things like "Beauty has always been dangerous" and "Women are willing to put up with it" — for instance, "Botox, let's stick frog poison in our eyebrows." He reminded me that the most common injury from cosmetics is getting poked in the eye with a mascara wand while driving. And he is especially skeptical of regulations because "it's a free country."

But when it comes to a safer cosmetics industry, Bruce is unequivocal: "We can do better. There are a lot of things in the world we can improve without too much work and this is one of them." Fragrances are "full of nasty molecules," according to Bruce, and in his opinion there is no excuse ever to use phthalates. However, he doesn't buy the idea that all personal care products should be made with food-grade ingredients and no chemicals at all. Certain synthetic chemicals such as bubble-making surfactants and emulsifiers, which help mix oil and water, give products the characteristics consumers have come to expect. However, there are safer choices companies can make within these chemical classes.

Formulating cosmetics is "not rocket science," just six to eight hours in a lab that any of us could do, according to Bruce. Twenty to 30 chemicals make up the core of most products, and certain essential ingredients are problematic from a toxicity standpoint. For instance, preservatives: since it's their job to kill bacteria, preservatives are typically toxic. "Until companies want to ship stuff cold and people are willing to take it home and treat it like perishables, you can't get rid of preservatives," Bruce explained. Everyone agrees that parabens are cheap and effective preservatives, but the chemicals are also estrogenic and persistent. In recent years, many natural products companies have switched to alternative preservatives, using mixtures of benzoic acid, sorbic acid and bezyl alcohol, among other chemicals.

To get the safest products, consumers ultimately may have to change some expectations. "When you walk into a room, does *everybody* really need to smell you? People have to get away from the idea that that's what perfume is," Bruce said. "Someone close to you can smell it, but don't leave it in an elevator for half an hour." Likewise, products may not need a three-year shelf life, and of course, the safest products are not likely to be the cheapest — at least not until safe ingredients become the norm. "Safer, high-quality products cost more to make, but companies will make them if they understand people care about that," Bruce explained simply. "It will take people demanding, 'We're not buying this crap'."

## Tween Beauty

How do you get young girls to see behind the glossy ads to their own natural beauty? You wouldn't expect a young man in his early 20s to be pondering such a problem. But when his sister turned 9, Max Ritzenberg and his stepmom Stacey Cooper decided to launch a new company called Tween Beauty, as "a driver to spread the word" to pre-teenage girls about safe ingredients and the true meaning of beauty.

"At that age there's so much being pushed down their throats about society's idea of beauty — of outer beauty, and having a body like a model and having a painted face. We did not want that to be our idea of beauty," Max said, so they chose to sell hair products and body wash rather than makeup. "We decided beauty was cleanliness and being confident in yourself and being excited about how you look, not because you look like a model but because you wear clothes that express your style, and you wear your hair in a way that expresses yourself and makes you feel good about yourself," explained Max. "Beauty is doing well in school, and beauty is excelling in the activities that you like, and beauty is hanging out with your friends and feeling good about yourself."

It's a big idea to package in a bottle, but the girls helped figure it out. Max's sister and her friends, more than a dozen girls age 7 to 12, chose the package designs and product scents. "We worked really hard to make our product just as cool, smell just as great if not better and work just as well as any alternative," Max said. "It's important because that age group is so trend driven and so conscious of what their peers are using and the celebrities are using. They weren't going to choose shampoo in a boring green bottle. If you really want to hook them early, your products have to be better than synthetic alternatives. The girls have to choose our products because they're the best products, because they love them the most, and then once they love our products, we educate them that natural can be cool — that natural is even more cool."

Max talks about natural products with the enthusiasm of an evangelist and the precision of an A student who has done his homework. "When I started this company, it wasn't that one day I said we need to stop poisoning our children. I really didn't know anything about cosmetics or toxins," Max recalled. But then, "I started reading about all the toxins and all these horrible ingredients making their way into these products, and I started reading about the approval process for cosmetics, which is stunning. There is no approval process basically —

anybody can bottle anything and put it on the shelf and call it whatever they want to."

To learn about product ingredients, Max ordered books on cosmetic chemistry, read scientific studies from *Pub Med* and scoured the Internet for information from reliable sources. "There's contradictory information all over the place. You have to have a discerning eye for what's legit and what's not," Max said. "Some of these are suspected," he commented, referring to toxic ingredients suspected of causing health problems although there is no proof. "But when you're looking at something that has long-term implications, something that's a carcinogen that wouldn't show up as cancerous cells for 20 to 30 years, why use it? Why include it in your daily regimen?" Max wonders why, instead of addressing problems at the source, we try to fix them at the back end. Why don't we work on preventing cancer, instead of just treating it? "Prevention has got to be somebody's priority."

Max compared starting a company to the prospect of raising a child. "You want to raise it with these principles and ideals, and it can't just be one thing. You can't just say it's important to use safe natural cosmetics. It's also important to understand the importance of biodegradability and recycling, and eating healthy and organic foods when possible, and drinking milk without hormones, and it just spreads to everything. It was imperative to make sure that everything we did with the company was in line with our principles, with what we wanted to contribute to society, not only inside the bottles but outside."

## Back to the Future

"This is an industry that is in many ways a laboratory for social change," said Morris Shriftman, a natural products salesman for more than 30 years, and current vice president of marketing for Avalon Organics.[6] The industry has been through three waves of reform, according to Morris. "The first reform was food," and involved cleaning up food ingredients and shifting the way people think about meat. The second reform asked "Why does agriculture have to use so many toxic, synthetic, persistent, dangerous chemicals? Do we really need all that?" This led to the organic food standards. "In the third reform, we asked the same questions about skin care, cosmetics and body care products. Why do these products have to have so many objectionable ingredients? And that takes us to Consciousness in Cosmetics."

The phrase refers to his company's recent efforts to reformulate products in response to the Compact for Safe Cosmetics. Morris explained the history of Avalon's change of consciousness. "We got to know Jeanne [Rizzo] and all the people up there at the Breast Cancer Fund and really developed a very strong appreciation and respect for them and for their work, and it was an eye-opener for us," Morris explained. "We decided that there was something that we could do as a company to support that work and redefine the notion of safety, purity and efficacy in personal care products. We looked at every ingredient in our products and saw that there were opportunities for us to improve."

Over the next year, the company spent about $1 million to reformulate more than 100 products, according to Morris, eliminating phthalates, formaldehyde donors and some petroleum-based ingredients. They added new organic ingredients and a new baby-product line. ("When you see some of the baby skin care on the market you wonder, how the hell are these products still on the market?" Morris observed.)

In a move that ignited a brief firestorm of controversy in the natural products industry, Avalon also removed parabens preservatives and advertised their products "parabens free" — thus putting the spotlight on an ingredient many competitors were using. Tensions boiled to the surface at the 2005 Natural Products Expo West at a panel about the Campaign for Safe Cosmetics. During the Q&A session, angry questions flew at Morris Shriftman. What was Avalon using instead of parabens? Why wouldn't they share the formula for the alternative preservatives? How did they know the alternatives were safer? As the voices grew louder, Avalon CEO Gil Pritchard stood up from the middle of the crowd and addressed the room in a booming, very CEO-like voice. Avalon was just trying to do the right thing, he said, and if they didn't like it, tough. He said the company would share their information about alternatives with anyone else who wanted to get out of parabens.

Morris has no regrets. "To the allegation or the claim that we did that as a marketing device to differentiate ourselves from the competition, the answer is, yes we did," he said. "But was that the only reason? No. We wanted to establish a new standard for our industry and create a level of respect that will lift the whole natural products industry." Parabens are "insidious" in his opinion. "We decided that there was enough data on the danger of parabens for us to adopt the precautionary principle and eliminate them," though it wasn't an easy decision to switch out an effective ingredient. "People thought we were crazy to do that."

There were initial difficulties — problems with products separating on the shelves and product returns, as well as challenges working with manufacturers who had to learn to do things differently — "but it's all been worth it," Morris said, "because now our manufacturers have an unbelievably diverse experience and a capability they didn't have before … They have a different understanding of the impact of these ingredients on health, and they are now in mission alignment with us in this campaign for safe cosmetics."

There are hopeful signs in the laboratory for social change, but also challenges — for instance, a distribution system that is rigged against smaller companies. Retail stores make various demands of manufacturers: slotting allowances, "free fills," free samples, free demos, "ship us a case of 12 and we'll pay 10," Morris explained. "Basically what they're telling you is, look, in order to put your products on the shelf, we have to take something off. And what we're taking off could be a product that could theoretically sell more, or is selling more, than what you could sell. We have a risk, but we're willing to take that risk if you'll mitigate it." Big companies such as Procter & Gamble can more easily absorb the costs, and also have close relationships with buyers. A company like Avalon could wait months to see a retail buyer whereas P&G can get an appointment on a minute's notice, according to Morris.

As more consumers become interested in natural products, there is also the trend of large companies co-opting the message. Morris offered the example of Clairol Herbal Essence. "Their theme line is 'the organic experience' — very smart. What's organic about their products? I don't know. I'd say not too much, but Clairol Herbal Essence probably, as a product line, does more in sales than all of the natural products companies in personal care put together." He was quick to add: "I'm trying not to be judgmental because you know different companies have different values and do things differently. But it's a question of how you handle new knowledge."

Upon learning about the European Union Cosmetics Directive and the growing concerns about toxic ingredients, "We had one reaction to new knowledge, and that was, how can we use this new knowledge in the most productive way?" Morris said. "But a lot of companies, and a lot of individuals, resist new knowledge. They resist change. They're afraid of change. They want to delay it. They want to postpone it. They want to make believe they didn't hear anything."

Now in the midst of its third wave, the natural products industry has bright prospects ahead. "The message of natural products is breaking through to mainstream culture, there's no question about it," Morris said. "As more consumers become aware of the chemicals in their products and the chemical soup we're living in in general, they will see value in natural and organic." The reforms are a work in progress. "There's always new knowledge," Morris noted. Those who are willing to rise to the challenge, incorporate new knowledge and drive the market toward responsible choices are on the "hero's journey," he said. "In many ways we are all together in what can only be called a quest, a mission toward the improvement of life."

## Writing the Future

By January 2007, more than 500 companies had signed the Compact for Safe Cosmetics, agreeing to replace ingredients linked to cancer, birth defects, hormone disruption and other negative health effects with safer alternatives. Compact signers include big names such as Burt's Bees, Kiss My Face and Aubrey Organics as well as many smaller natural product manufacturers.[7] Notably absent are the world's largest cosmetics companies, the brands that fill the shelves in most drugstores and high-end specialty stores across the US and Canada — L'Oréal, Revlon, Estée Lauder (its subsidiary Aveda), Avon, Mary Kay, Procter & Gamble and their brands. For the time being, the big-name companies seem wedded to using the "same old soap technologies" and spending their resources on marketing campaigns to convince consumers their products are safe.

The Campaign for Safe Cosmetics, meanwhile, faces the challenge of how to make the Compact pledge meaningful in the world — how to track company compliance and how to define safer ingredients in a landscape where there are so many unknowns about the health impacts of chemicals. The huge response to the Compact was a "be careful what you wish for phenomenon," said Janet Nudelman of the Breast Cancer Fund. "Not exactly a monster, but a challenge." Her phone was ringing off the hook with questions and requests from Compact-signing companies. "We extended this pretty hefty challenge to the cosmetics industry as articulated by the Compact for Safe Cosmetics. Quite honestly, we've pulled many of them into a brand-new conversation, and we have to provide them with the tools to do what we've asked them to do," Janet explained. "It's just proven to be a really interesting challenge and a really big, big piece of work. We're really going down this path together, and I feel like we're partners in this work."

It's a creative challenge that the founding mother of the Campaign for Safe Cosmetics never imagined back when she was laying sticky notes on a conference table in the summer of 2002, trying to save the *Not Too Pretty* report from ending up in the dust bin. "Rather than being in a simple, predictable single-plot story, we're all in a novel together, and we're writing it one chapter at a time," Charlotte Brody told the 40 company representatives gathered at a meeting of Compact signers in the fall of 2006. "We know what we want at the end: to define safe in a way that means safe for everyone over the long term. And to make things safer every year, so at the end of the novel we actually come out with healthier people and babies born toxic-free. That's a novel worth writing."

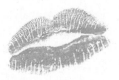

# 11

# The Face of the Future:
## Green Chemistry, Green Politics

How to make plywood kitchen cabinets without using glue made of cancer-causing formaldehyde? Dr. Kaichang Li was pondering the problem as he walked along Oregon's Cannon Beach. An alternative glue would need to be water resistant, strong, inexpensive — easy to make, like urea formaldehyde, only without the alarming toxicity — Dr. Li was thinking as he gazed out at the ocean, settling into a state of semi-attention. Suddenly, his eyes focused on the answer right in front of him: tiny mussels, clinging tenaciously to a rock in the crashing waves. These creatures knew how to be sticky.

Dr. Li scraped a few mussels off the rock and took them back to his lab at Oregon State University, where he works as a wood science professor. He studied the mussels' adhesive substance and replicated it with a protein-based resin made from soy flour. The result: non-toxic, water-soluble, cost-effective glue that works perfectly for making plywood kitchen cabinets. "Back to nature" is taking on a whole new meaning in today's material economy.

## Secrets from the Wild
"Nature doesn't scrub up with detergents," pointed out Janine Benyus, who wrote the book on epiphanies from the natural world, *Biomimicry: Innovation Inspired by Nature*.[1] Biomimicry — the imitation of biological

organisms — is a new science that analyzes nature's best ideas and adapts them to human use. The idea is that after billions of years of evolution, the natural world has already figured a few things out: how to manufacture waterproof fiber five times stronger than steel (spiders), convert sunlight into fuel in trillionths of a second (leaves), create color by refracting light (peacocks). The answers to human technological "problems," in other words, are living all around us.

Janine Benyus talks about nature's teachings with a reverence that makes you want to go out and befriend a butterfly. Biomimicry seeks to build new relationships with the natural world by using nature's wisdom to design human activities. On the topic of cleaning, for instance, just ask the experts in the field. "We tend to think of the natural world as being dirty, but in fact there is a great need for organisms to stay clean. Cleaning is a survival issue," Janine explained. Leaves need to stay free of debris in order to feed themselves with the sun. Oaks have devised an excellent strategy: their leaves are covered with tiny hairs that work like fine bristles to keep debris off the pores underneath. The "hairy leaf strategy" could be borrowed for human products such as clothes or buildings. "Instead of making buildings with little hairy buffers, we think about sandblasting them once they get dirty," Janine reflected. "We don't think preventatively, but these organisms do."

From her office in Montana where she runs the Biomimicry Guild, a consulting firm for companies seeking nature-inspired design ideas, Janine Benyus took me through a slide show of colorful creatures with various cleaning strategies. "Nowhere in the natural world do we have soaps and surfactants used to clean. It's not one of the mechanisms life uses," Janine explained. "Life either resists dirt or doesn't get dirty to begin with." There are mechanical approaches (eyelids), structural solutions (the hairy leaf) and chemical applications (mucous or saliva) — but "none of those things are toxic."

One structural strategy with commercial applicability is the Lotus Effect — "the next Velcro," as Janine called it. Lotus leaves are covered with nano-sized bumps like a bed of tiny, waxy nails.[2] Dirt stays loose on the tips of the bumps, then rainwater balls up and sweeps the dirt away. Self-cleaning paint modeled on the Lotus Effect is already being used on 300,000 homes in Europe. "Why is self-cleaning built into the structure so that the organism doesn't have to use extra chemicals? Because that's expensive. In the natural world, the rewards and spoils go to the organism that can make the material itself the system, without the extra stuff," Benyus said. "My answer to you about cleaning is: don't get dirty in the first place." The cosmetics industry, she suggested, should look to self-cleaning and self-healing products for its future: "maybe coating hair with something that helps dirt slide off it — a structural rather than chemical solution."

## Buzz Worthy Curls

Structural solutions for hair treatment may seem far-fetched, but they're already happening. Half a continent away in her lab at the University of Massachusetts, Lowell, Amy Cannon has devised just such a strategy for curling and coloring hair. Cannon holds the world's first PhD in green chemistry, a science that designs chemical products and processes in ways that reduce or eliminate hazardous substances. Her recent project involved using UV light to shrink-wrap hair into a non-toxic perm. The concept, known as "water-soluble photocrosslinking materials in cosmetics," won the Society of Cosmetic Chemists' award for best paper in 2006.[3] Dozens of chemists lined up to talk to Cannon after she presented the idea at the society's annual meeting. They told her it was the most innovative thing they'd seen in cosmetic chemistry in a long time.

Not bad for an idea that started out as a joke. "We were having lunch with two undergrads to talk about plate tectonics … and we started talking about the hair gel viscosity in Dippity-do," explained John Warner, PhD, director of the green chemistry program at UMass Lowell and co-author of the award-winning paper. The students were developing a new super-thin, water-based polymer that gets sticky when exposed to ultraviolet light. Maybe we should try it in hair, someone suggested. We could shape the hair into a curl, dip it in the polymer and shrinkwrap it into a non-toxic perm. Regular hair perming technologies, in contrast, work by reducing and oxidizing the hair itself. "It's some of the most toxic chemistry out there in the synthetic lab, never mind putting it on your hair," Amy Cannon explained.

The students, thinking the whole thing was funny, put together a PowerPoint presentation as a joke. One day, John Warner was giving a presentation to a large corporation (which he declines to name, though it's not a cosmetics firm) and "decided to be an amusing person and show them this amusing slide show." As he explained the non-toxic perm, he noticed a couple executives in the audience get up and leave the room, looking quite serious. They later cornered him and said the non-toxic perm idea was "the most innovative thing we've ever heard of in hair technology."

Imagine similar innovations everywhere in the material economy. Imagine safe chemistry in the lab; non-polluting chemical factories in communities; non-toxic cosmetics, plastics and furniture in our homes. "This is about everything we see, touch and hold in our hats," according to Paul Anastas, PhD, the father of green chemistry and former director of the US EPA Green Chemistry Program. "There is a new scientific awareness. We don't just know *that* something is toxic, we know why it happens. This allows scientists now to design substances at the molecular level so that they do not induce toxic effects," Anastas said.

In 1998, Anastas and John Warner devised the "12 principles of green chemistry," a framework for designing inherently safer chemicals.[4] "The moment a chemist puts pencil to paper, he or she is making decisions about human health and environmental impacts. Chemists bring new things into the world and design them to have certain properties," Anastas explained. "They manipulate things to be blue or red, soft or brittle. In the same way, they can design things to be safe or hazardous." A chemist could, for instance, design a dye that is not only red, but also non-carcinogenic and biodegradable. Or she could design a non-toxic polymer that is inherently red in the first place and needs no extra dye.

Similar to the biomimicry lesson about self-cleaning strategies, green chemistry seeks to build the desired functionality into molecules at the beginning of the design process rather than adding molecules later — the fewer expensive additions, the better. Amy Cannon's light-reactive polymer, for example, is inherently flexible so it doesn't require extra plasticizers that could shed off or leach out into people's bodies. A diabolically opposite example is vinyl plastic: the material is produced with hazardous materials, contributes cancer-causing dioxin to the air during the manufacturing process, and requires the addition of toxic stabilizers (lead) and plasticizers (phthalates) to make it soft and flexible for consumer products like lunchboxes and yellow rubber duckies.

Looking around the living room — the office, kitchen or kids' playroom — one can see no shortage of toxic products that could be redesigned or replaced with safer green chemistry alternatives. According to John Warner, "Of all the chemical products and processes out there in the universe, about 10% are benign and nontoxic; 90% of things we're doing today in 2006 have hazardous consequences." Of those toxic materials, Warner estimates that 25% could be replaced relatively easily with existing safer alternatives. "But the other 65%? Today we do not have solutions to provide to industry. The current way we have chemistry set up does not even touch these needs."

Warner wants to know: who's going to invent the replacement technologies? Astonishingly, no university in the United States requires chemists to demonstrate knowledge about the health and environmental impacts of the chemicals they create — not one. According to John Warner, even PhD chemists are not required to take courses in toxicology, biology or environmental health. Only a handful of schools in the US teach green chemistry at all. "People say there's nothing new to invent," Warner laments. "This is a whole new area for innovation, for creativity, for cutting-edge technology. It's a huge opportunity."

So what's the holdup? Human nature? Fear of change? Entrenched industries? Entrenched academia? All of the above. Warner blames a myopic academic system focused on high productivity, published results and federal grants that encourage students to think in silos and not look at the broader implications of their work. Old-guard chemistry professors are suspicious of new approaches. "Science changes one funeral at a time," as the saying goes. Another problem: chemistry programs are already packed full of requirements; adding a green chemistry or toxicology course would mean eliminating something else. (Warner suggests axing the requirement to translate scientific papers into French, since computer programs can do that nowadays.) Chemistry accreditation requirements are set by the American Chemical Society, which is largely funded by major chemical, pharmaceutical and product manufacturers — companies that would, presumably, find ways to profit from safer, less-polluting green chemistry technologies.

It's the Great Green Paradox: At a time when global demand is rising for green industries, the United States is investing few resources in green chemistry and clean technologies, and there are few scientists in the pipeline to fill the need. "What's needed is no less than a fundamental cultural shift," according to Paul Anastas. America needs a new environmental mindset — one that focuses on designing safer products at the front end rather than trying to clean up the pollution at the back end. "In order to get there, we need to make greener more economically profitable, so what is better for health and the environment is also better for the competitive advantage," Anastas said. Green chemistry is conceptually straightforward, he said, but not scientifically easy. "What we have is a great scientific challenge. We're on the first step of a thousand mile journey, a journey of continuous innovation. It's not that we can't do it, but will we embrace this at the level of urgency that is necessary to make this change?"

## The Politics of Falling Behind

What's also needed is a fundamental shift in American politics. Case in point: your kitchen cabinets. Why — if Dr. Kaichang Li has already invented a non-toxic, cost-effective replacement for urea formaldehyde — do most new kitchen cabinets sold in the US let off formaldehyde gas? The majority of plywood cabinets sold in US stores come from China, but it's not that Chinese factories aren't already making formaldehyde-free cabinets and furniture. They are; it's just that they're shipping the less-toxic products to Japan and Europe while the US market gets the formaldehyde.

Japan and Europe — even China itself — restrict formaldehyde in wood furniture products due to health concerns. But the US has no federal limits on formaldehyde in consumer products, so cabinets in schools and homes across the nation can contain unlimited amounts of the cancer-causing chemical. The California Air Resources Board (CARB) restricted formaldehyde in the spring of 2007, although the rules give companies until 2009 to make safer products that are already required in Europe. At a recent CARB hearing, dozens of furniture manufacturers testified that formaldehyde limits would reduce their profits and drive up consumer prices. The largest US manufacturer of plywood furniture disagrees. The Oregon-based Columbia Forest Products is already making formaldehyde-free plywood cabinets using Dr. Li's mussel-inspired technology. After an initial up-front cost to switch the production facilities, the cost of manufacturing the safer glue is about the same, according to the company's public relations manager John McIsaac.

"We know it's not going to kill anybody's business [to eliminate formaldehyde]. We're living proof of that," McIsaac said. His company is pushing for strict standards in California, but the standards have grown weaker as other companies have lobbied against them. "It's kind of offensive to me because I know a lot of these people are already making products that are formaldehyde free. They just don't want to convert all their processes because they would have to make an investment. The rest of the industry needs to get on board with this! It's frustrating."

## American Beauty?

It's not just the formaldehyde cabinets. Like Columbia Forest Products, many US companies are interested in safer technologies but have a hard time competing with companies that aren't making those investments and that aren't required to inform consumers that their products contain harmful chemicals. Meanwhile, European companies are being pushed to develop safer technologies faster than their US counterparts. "While our government remains indifferent, the European Union has launched a long-term strategy for industrial transformation — nothing less," wrote William Greider in the *Nation*. "The EU is forcing industry, sector by sector, to undertake the redesign of products, production processes and packaging." [5]

Americans are getting left in the toxic dust, quite literally. "As the European Union and other nations have tightened their environmental standards, mostly in the last two years, manufacturers ... are selling goods to American consumers that fail to meet other nations' stringent laws for toxic chemicals," reported Marla Cone in the *Los Angeles Times*. "Wood, toys, electronics, pesticides and cosmetics are among US products that contain substances that are banned or restricted elsewhere, particularly in Europe and Japan, because they may raise the risk of cancer, alter hormones or cause reproductive or neurological damage." [6]

Guided by the precautionary principle, the European Union is requiring manufacturers to eliminate toxins and take responsibility for the waste they create. In contrast, the United States is guided by a "prove harm" approach. The Environmental Protection Agency must prove a toxic substance "presents an unreasonable risk of injury to health or the environment" before regulating it — which roughly translates to "show us the dead bodies." The burden of proof is so high that the EPA hasn't even been able to ban certain uses of asbestos, and hasn't even tried to ban a toxic compound since it lost the asbestos fight in court 18 years ago. Under the weak US regulatory system, industrial chemicals are allowed onto the market with little or no health and safety data, consumer products can contain unlimited amounts of toxic chemicals, and there is no way for consumers or businesses to tell the difference between safe and hazardous products.

"In the market we have created through our public policies, there is no pressing need for companies to design their products to be as safe as possible," said Michael P. Wilson, PhD, a research scientist at the University of California, Berkeley. In a report to the California legislature, Wilson and his coauthors recommended that the state create new chemical policies that shift the market toward green chemistry. Otherwise, the state will face growing environmental and health problems and risk being left behind in the global economy.[7]

"Our universities are not teaching green chemistry because industry isn't demanding chemists with this kind of knowledge," Wilson said. "The fact is that innovating new products, from both a technical and commercial viability point of view, is very difficult to do. The process of innovation is expensive and uncertain. Companies are motivated to invest in new products only if they are fairly certain a market will be there. Public policies are needed to get the market working properly so consumers and businesses can confidently choose safer substances." Just as California's energy-efficiency policies have fostered a vibrant solar industry in the state, effective chemical policies would likewise birth new industries in green chemistry and clean manufacturing to meet the demands of the 21st-century global economy.

Learn more about the efforts to reform state and national efforts to phase out hazardous chemicals and shift the market toward safer green chemistry alternatives.
chemicalspolicy.org

## New Year, New You

"All we have to do is design new systems. That's new business," as Aveda's creator Horst Rechelbacher told cosmetics industry CEOs in Miami. You might think the cosmetics industry — the billion-dollar makers of chemical-containing products we routinely apply to our bodies — would be at the front of the line investing in research to create the next generation of safer chemicals. The problem is, old systems die hard. "Cosmetics companies are very careful in their formulation changes, more so than other industries," said UC Berkeley's Michael Wilson. "People get used to formulas, and for most products there are no obvious short-term health effects. If a company has a product that is working, it's going to be really difficult to move them off of that product on arguments around toxicity unless you do it through regulation."

It's not that consumers don't value safe cosmetics, judging by the number of beauty ads that emphasize the words *healthy, clean, pure* and *natural.* But with no standards in the industry, the commercial advantage goes to companies that spend the most money on ads to convince consumers their products are pure — regardless of what's actually in them.

There's no shortage of possibilities for green cosmetic chemistry innovation, in chemist Amy Cannon's view. Nail polish, for instance: pigments, solvents, dispersants, stabilizers, plasticizers and resins all present opportunities for reform. Could resin be made inherently sticky, thereby eliminating the need for plasticizers? Maybe we could check in with the peacocks; they've already figured out how to create brilliant colors by refracting light through a matrix of keratin, the same substance human fingernails are made of. "Why are we still talking about chemicals and paint? Why don't you just design thin layers that play with light?" asked Janine Benyus of the Biomimicry Guild. The super-thin photosensitive polymer Amy Cannon developed for hair perms may also be applicable to hair color with a coating of food-grade dye. But then, Amy's got classes to teach, and there's little financial support coming her way for work on cosmetics.

"If we do not change our direction, we are likely to end up where we are headed," as the ancient Chinese proverb goes. The story of chemistry brings us to a fork in the road. The petrochemical infrastructure of the mid 20th century — designed for function and convenience, with little thought to safety and health — is a relic of times when we could believe humans were somehow separate from the toxic systems we created. Now we know: the chemical poisons that run through rivers, fish and polar bears are running through the umbilical cord to our children. The carcinogen in the baby shampoo can't be separated from the carcinogens in the food and the air, just as the polluting chemical plants aren't separate from the leaching trash dumps at the end of the line; they aren't separate from the skyrocketing asthma rates or the chemo parties in the brand-new children's cancer ward.

The story of chemistry also brings us to the threshold of new possibilities. Designing substances at the molecular level so they do not induce toxic effects — who ever thought chemistry could be so cool! Green chemistry is the recipe for the next industrial revolution, the building block for a new carbon-neutral, toxic-free, zero-waste green economy that lives in harmony with the natural world. "Running the economy like a redwood forest," as Janine Benyus describes it. The mature redwood system knows how to do more with less; it reuses materials over and over, recycles every single thing and lives in synergy with the species around it, recognizing that every part of the system is a part of itself.

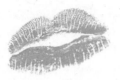

# 12

## *Extreme Makeover*

The women went to the Dow Chemical Company shareholder meeting carrying 5,000 brooms and chemical-contaminated soil from their hometown. "In India, the broom is a woman's symbol of power. Being struck by a *jhadoo* (broom) is the ultimate insult," explained Champi Devi Shukla. "By delivering *jhadoos* to Dow, we're telling the company to clean up its mess in Bhopal."

Two decades after a chemical plant meltdown sent 27 tons of toxic gas into their sleeping city, the women of Bhopal, India, are leading the fight to bring justice to their people and to remind the world about the worst face of the chemical revolution. "Mothers everywhere in the world carry chemical poisons in their breasts," said Rashida Bee as she accepted the 2004 Goldman Environmental Prize with Shukla for their efforts in Bhopal. "We are not expendable. We are not flowers offered at the altar of profit and power. We are dancing flames committed to conquering darkness and to challenging those who threaten the planet and the magic and mystery of life." [1]

Women have long been flames at the forefront of the fight for environmental health and justice: from Rachel Carson, who exposed the dangers of pesticides and launched the modern environmental movement with her brave book *Silent Spring;* to Lois Gibbs and the families of Love Canal, who put human faces and stories to the "someplace else" of chemical waste dumps; to the women of Bhopal and thousands of others around the world who are fighting to clean up dangerously contaminated communities. Women have long borne the brunt of pollution and poverty. Yet today, more women have more power than ever before. As the primary shoppers and the largest block of voters in the United States, women can shift the balance of power and change the face of the future.

"We are the ones we have been waiting for," as the poet June Jordan said, and as Alice Walker affirmed in the title of her recent book. "It is the best of times," Walker wrote, "because we have entered a period, if we can bring ourselves to pay attention, of great clarity as to cause and effect." [2] We know now that the environment is us — it is our wombs, our breast milk and our families. Protecting the environment is about enabling future generations of our children to thrive in unpolluted bodies.

There is so much cleaning up to do. The problem right in front of our faces, the toxic products on the bathroom sink, is a place to start. First cosmetics then on to the next cleanup project: the plastic industry, the petrochemical industry, the oil and war industries too — until there are no more toxic chemicals in babies, rocket fuel in breast milk, or communities burdened by toxic pollution; until we create new economic systems that are compatible with life and healthy for people and the planet. Each better choice is a step on the road to getting there. Here are some ideas for giving the cosmetics industry a makeover.

## Girlcotts — Choosing Safer, Kinder Products

"The simpler the better," was Dr. Devra Davis's shopping advice for choosing safer personal care products. With all the new data about cosmetic ingredients that has emerged in the past several years, I keep going back to that four-word sentence as one of the most important take-away messages. Simpler products, fewer ingredients, fewer unknown and unnecessary products and ingredients — that's the gist of my personal shopping guidelines. Like Laura Jones, the former makeup diva who off-loaded her silver tackle box of high-end products, I too have switched to a small canvas bag of products that don't smell like a synthetic chemistry lab. As an added bonus, a few months after I switched to natural shampoo, my skin cleared up. Some other simple shopping rules on my list: no synthetic "fragrance," no estrogenic ingredients such as parabens or placenta, and no false advertising claims of "pure and gentle" products that may be contaminated with carcinogens. These few guidelines, unfortunately, eliminate many personal care products on the shelves of mainstream stores.

I don't think of it as a boycott, exactly — more like a "girlcott," which was another idea offered by Devra Davis. "Boycotts mean saying no. Girlcotts mean yes," Dr. Davis explained. "Women are the main purchasers of products and take responsibility for what goes into the home. We can organize to change market forces by saying we don't want cancer-causing products and we do want safer products. When enough women get together, we can make things happen."

## Keep it Simple:

- Eliminate unnecessary products — for instance bubble bath, especially for babies, is often a bath full of unwanted chemical exposures.
- Use your nose as a guide — after switching to natural products, I found the smell of synthetic fragrance to be less appealing; sort of like when you drink a diet cola after not drinking one for a while and immediately notice the chemical smell.
- Buy from companies you trust — many companies have high standards for ingredient safety, good social values and effective products; investigating the companies themselves rather than just the ingredients can be a simpler way to choose the best products.
- Start with high-exposure, frequently used products — shampoo, face cream, deodorant and other products used in larger amounts. Lip and hand products that can be ingested are good products to switch first.

A note about standardized labeling: some companies, particularly European ones, use standardized labeling (called INCI) that requires chemical rather than natural names of ingredients. The INCI standards are good labeling practice, and ingredients are often explained in further detail on product labels or company websites.

Find safer products:

- SafeCosmetics.org
- ResponsiblePurchasing.org
- LessToxicGuide.ca
- BigGreenPurse.com
- TheNakedTruthProject.org
- GreenLivingNow.com
- Safer-Products.org

It's fun to think about spending my money on the kind of world I want to create. *Yes* to women finding and celebrating true beauty in ourselves and in each other; *no* to computerized skin tones and wrinkle-erased beauty ads. *No* to an organic experience created in a petrochemical factory. *No*, I don't want to invest in a vision of the future that involves selling skin whitening cream to millions of villages in China. *Yes* to products that are safe for the fish, the frogs and all the species of the planet. *Yes* to cosmetics that are 100% free of toxic chemicals linked to birth defects, cancer and learning disabilities. *Yes* to gathering together in communities and building political power to change the rules so that any of us can go into any store, any time, and buy any personal care products without having to worry about whether they are safe for our families.

## Girls Get Together — Creating Political Space

Women build power by building networks of relationships — organizing like a girl, as Charlotte Brody called it. Cindy Luppi decided to throw in some natural products made from scratch. "It's been trial and error," explained Cindy, project director of the Boston-based group Clean Water Action. The first "Healthy Cosmetics Spa Party" she organized was a Halloween-themed party with products made from online recipes. "Some of them don't give a lot of directions," she found — for instance, the cranberry lip gloss that didn't say how long to cook the cranberry and ended up running down people's faces. "I haven't had the guts to try that again." She's had much better luck with Strawberry Sea Salt Hand and Foot Scrub, which "smells like summer, feels great and is a good group-building exercise."

Cindy's group has organized 50 spa parties in the New England area in the past couple years, bringing together some 500 people from labor unions, teachers' groups, religious communities and even state legislators to learn about toxic products and safer alternatives. "It's a way to bring women together and create a group bonding, and also to relate the cosmetics issue back to the larger political fight," Cindy explained. Some groups have

What's in that Make-up?
Cosmeticdatabase.org
ScoreCard.org
atsdr.cdc.gov/toxfaq.html
toxnet.nlm.nih.gov

Just for the health of it:
• BeSafeNet.com
• HealthyChildHealthyWorld.org

taken their first political steps after the spa party, such as a gathering of Chinese Americans that included 30 women, men and kids and an interpreter, all of whom wrote letters to legislators to support a bill to phase out mercury-containing products. "It was a really cool and powerful moment. The bill eventually passed and the group felt empowered by that." The Alliance for a Healthy Tomorrow coalition in New England is currently lobbying for the Safer Alternatives Bill, which will set up an ongoing program to replace harmful chemicals with safer alternatives.

Learn More:
HealthyTomorrow.org
Take Action:
SafeCosmetics.org/action

## Dial a Company — or Start One

The companies are listening. The big brand-conscious companies do pay attention to phone calls, letters and consumer demands, especially when they come in multiples or with television cameras in tow. So it's important to contact companies directly (and sometimes publicly) if you have questions or concerns about a product, even though as we've found, you don't always get the straight answer. Some questions you could ask

- What is the company doing to ensure its products aren't contaminated with 1,4-dioxane, formaldehyde, lead or other toxins not listed on labels?
- What chemicals are contained in the "fragrance"?
- Do their products contain phthalates (THA-lates) that aren't listed on the label? Although many products no longer contain dibutyl phthalate, many mainstream companies still use other types of phthalates in their products.
- Does the company have a substitution plan to identify hazardous ingredients and replace them with safer alternatives?
- Did they sign the Compact for Safe Cosmetics pledge?
- Is the company investing in green chemistry research and development?

## Paint the Town Green

Just about every profession and institution in sight could use a green makeover: schools, hospitals, cities. You name it, you can green it. While individuals can wield only so much power, institutions with major buying clout can shift the market instantaneously. As one example, when Kaiser Permanente, the largest nonprofit health care system in the US, decided to purchase PVC-free materials for new construction, a carpet manufacturer agreed to develop a new PVC-free product made with non-toxic, recycled plastic at no extra cost. In exchange, the vendor won an exclusive contract with the health care system to supply carpet for millions of square feet in new construction. "In an era of rising construction costs, you don't have to pay extra money and use precious healthcare dollars just to be green," Christine Malcolm, a vice president at Kaiser Permanente, told the *Wall Street Journal*.[3] With the industry's purchasing power, "we can force suppliers to generate environmentally sensitive products." Major institutions, government agencies and entire industries can create markets for non-toxic products and drive down costs for bio-based plastics, green chemistry, renewable energy and other solutions for the future. The billion-dollar cosmetics industry, of course, could be a major force for positive

Green...
Schools: GreenSchools.net
Hospitals: NoHarm.org
Buildings: HealthyBuilding.Net
Business: GreenGuide.com
Science: SEHN.org
Computers: ComputerTakeBack.com
News: EnvironmentalHealthNews.org

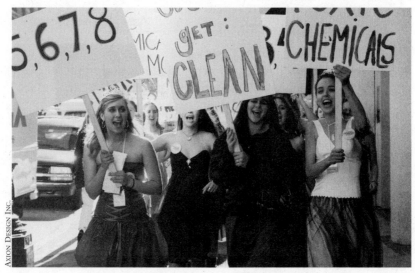

*Teens rally for safe cosmetics around Union Square in San Francisco.*

change if they were to seriously invest in green chemistry innovation and demand safer chemicals from the chemical industry.

## Giving the Government a Makeover

We can't just shop our way out of this problem. Jeremiah Holland and Michelle Hammond — the parents from Berkeley, California, who, along with their two children, were the first family to be biomonitored in the US — have had many conversations about the chemicals found in their bodies. For Jeremiah, there is one key message to get across: "I think the most important thing is to not assume that you're going to make any kind of a difference just by change in the market [shopping]. The only solution is to change public policy so these chemicals are banned at the point of production," he said. "Until that happens we're all guinea pigs. If it's in your nail polish, it's in my body. If it's in your mattress, it's in my body."

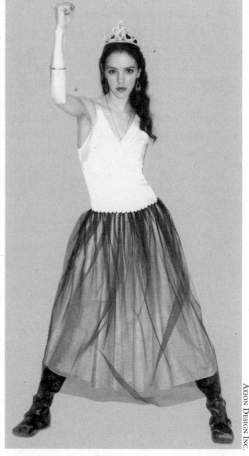

Some of Michelle's friends reacted to her story by joking that it was time to move to Idaho or some other remote location. "You can't move anywhere on the planet anymore to avoid this stuff," Michelle pointed out. "Even if you have all the safest products in your house, you open your window, your child goes to school. You can't stick your head in the sand and stick your little butt up in the air on this one. So get involved. Don't be scared. Just get involved in any way you can."

*Erin Schrode in a prom dress and combat boots to signify the teens' war on toxic chemicals, for the "Project Prom" rally in San Francisco's Union Square.*

AXION DESIGN INC.

From MOMS organizing to clean up their breast milk, to health care systems demanding safer products, to the forward-thinking governments around the world that are passing precautionary, health-protective chemical policies, momentum is building for change. "The chemical industry is also going to have to change. The world is changing," as Horst Rechelbacher said. The only question is, can we change it fast enough?

In the most hopeful of signs, the younger generation is taking up the torch. As high school junior Erin Schrode said as she stood onstage at Union Square dressed in a white prom dress and combat boots to signify the teenagers' war on toxic chemicals: "It's not just us who are affected but everyone around the world for generations to come. We can't change the environment singlehandedly, but we can certainly try, and in the process inspire others to do the same. This is simple. We must think tactically, know our facts, establish a strong platform, and pass laws to create change." Now that's a pink promise for the future worth making — sealed with a lead-free lipstick kiss.

# Epilogue

It's a sunny Sunday in Corte Madera, California, and the teens are sitting in a circle outside the mall. "We need to focus on getting girls signed up for the body burden testing. Think about the girls you know across the country — friends, relatives, friends of friends, and start networking," Judi Shils is saying, slouched back in her lawn chair. Around her neck, the silver "Search for the Cure" dog tags, etched with names of friends who have died of cancer, glint in the sunlight.

Today's agenda for the Teen Safe Cosmetics Campaign is ambitious: mini summits planned for San Francisco, Los Angeles and New York; a nationwide teen summit next February; a battle-of-the-bands benefit concert next month. Jessica Assaf, now a junior at Bransen Academy, unfurls the poster she drew for the benefit concert called Rock SAFE — for "Student Activists Feeling Empowered." Students will pay $10 each to see local bands compete for a chance to win $500 and studio recording time. Maybe they can also get the winning band on Alice radio station? That would be so cool! Jessica volunteers to ask the people at Alice. Does anyone have connections to famous people who could help with the concert? "I hear Pink's moving to Novato," says Kelly O'Boyle, from Marin Academy in San Rafael. "My friend's friend's father is a real estate agent who sold them a house."

Kelly joined the campaign a few months ago. "I'm learning all this stuff I had no idea about," she says. "All of the brands, even some of the ones that seem so earthy and stuff, are not at all." Jessica waves her hands excitedly. "I just had this vision," she says, eyes wide. Sweeping her hand in front of her, she describes a scene of 50,000 teenagers at Golden Gate Park, each paying $10 to see a Rock SAFE concert sponsored by Radio Alice with Pink kicking off the concert. "We could totally expand our campaign!" Judi is nodding, "Sort of like a teen Woodstock," she agrees, and then holds up her hand. "OK, OK, this is good. For once I'm being the grounded one," she says. First, they have to get a couple of hundred kids and some press coverage at Rock SAFE so the radio station can see the benefit of sponsoring a larger event next year. "Write up your vision," she tells Jessica.

The conversation turns to acne. Jessica is organizing a panel discussion for juniors and seniors. Many of her friends are taking birth control pills to clear up their skin or using harsh acne medications such as Acutane and Proactive. "What they don't know is the whole other side; they don't know how toxic these products are," Jessica says. She is bothered that doctors are prescribing the Pill "left right and sideways" as acne medication, even to girls as young as 12. She thinks there are healthier ways to deal with acne, such as diet improvements and natural skin remedies.

Three younger girls walk by. Katie Pilot, a freshman at Tamalpais High, jumps up and offers to take them over to the Green Spa, a tent just outside Banana Republic and the Gap, where the teens give free makeovers with natural products and spread the word about the safe cosmetics campaign. Katie returns to the meeting with good news: "The girls want a list of upcoming events; they're all excited. They want to do something right away." Ten minutes later, the girls walk by dressed in Teen Campaign for Safe Cosmetics apparel. "Look, look," Katie points. "They're wearing their new T-shirts, how cute!"

Katie is the epitome of cute herself. With polka-dotted shoes, sparkling eyes and the perfect pony tail, she could easily be one of America's Top Models, who are staring vacantly from every post outside the mall. But Katie has other things on her mind, and she offers a refreshing counterpoint to the messages of conformity and corporate-logo sameness that surround us. "I feel that, if companies are putting it out there, it should be safe. When you find out that there are so many things they don't tell you, it does scare you. I don't know one teen who, once I've told them about these different things, hasn't wanted to make a difference or know what they're putting on their face," Katie says. "If it's taken me this long to find out some of the truth behind makeup, you really want to make that information available to everyone."

To that end, Katie is volunteering two shifts at Green Spa, organizing girls in her school and helping publicize the safe cosmetics campaign. "I go where I'm needed," she says. "The nice thing is, it's real-life situations going on. It's great even to practice interviewing and talking to people. These are just different things you need in real life."

Katie speaks into my microphone as if she's done a hundred interviews. "Believe it or not, you can make a difference. By working together, we can accomplish something. I think that message isn't pushed enough with teens — that one person's idea, one person's thoughts, if you really are behind it, you can change something," she says. "And when I talk to people about getting involved, that's the number one thing I talk about. This is a chance to change something that needs to be dealt with, and you can make that change. It's not just that we're having adults, or the president or whoever — it's you, personally, changing something."

As Katie keeps talking, it feels like a new day is dawning right here at the mall. "I think it's just so great that kids are now finding out that they do have a choice and they can make positive choices for the better. When I really step back and think about it, this could be the start of something so big," says Katie, smiling brightly.

*Take Action:* SafeCosmetics.org
*Read the Toxic Beauty Blog for updates:* NotJustaPrettyFace.org

# Notes

## Prologue

1. Comment by Jared Blumenthal made onstage at "Project Prom," an outdoor rally in San Francisco's Union Square on April 7, 2007, organized by the Teen Campaign for Safe Cosmetics. All other quotes in subsequent chapters of the manuscript are based on personal interviews between March 2006 and April 2007 unless otherwise noted.

## Chapter 1

1. Jane Houlihan et al. "Body Burden: The Pollution in Newborns: A benchmark investigation of industrial chemicals, pollutants and pesticides in umbilical cord blood." Environmental Working Group, July 14, 2005.
2. June 2004 survey of 2,300 adults about personal care product use, conducted by the Environmental Working Group and Campaign for Safe Cosmetics.
3. Centers for Disease Control and Prevention. "National Report on Human Exposure to Environmental Chemicals." [online]. [cited May 4, 2007]. cdc.gov/exposurereport/. Also see Environmental Working Group. "Human Taxome Project: Mapping the Pollution in People." [online]. [cited May 4, 2007]. bodyburden.org.
4. The biomonitoring study led by Mount Sinai School of Medicine, Environmental Working Group and Commonweal in 2003 was the first to look for such a wide range of pollutants in the bodies of people from the general population. Charlotte was one of nine volunteers, including journalist Bill Moyers, who participated in the study. Jane Houlihan et al. "Body Burden: The Pollution in People." Environmental Working Group, January 2003.
5. Douglas Fischer. "What's in You?" *Oakland Tribune,* March 27, 2006. Part one of a three-part series. All parts of series can be viewed at "A Body's Burden: Our Chemical Legacy." [online]. [cited April 22, 2007]. insidebayarea.com/bodyburden.
6. Aake Bergman quoted in Fischer, note 5. Also see Douglas Fischer, "It's In Us All." *Oakland Tribune,* March 27, 2006.

7. National Academy of Sciences. "Pesticides in the Diets of Infants and Children." National Academy Press, 1993.
8. Peter Waldman. "Common Industrial Chemicals In Tiny Doses Raise Health Issue." *Wall Street Journal,* July 25, 2005.
9. Rachel Carson. *Silent Spring.* Houghton Mifflin, 1962.
10. See Lois Gibbs. "Learning from Love Canal: A 20th Anniversary Retrospective." [online]. [cited May 5, 2007]. *Orion Afield,* Spring 1998. arts.envirolink.org/arts_and_activism/LoisGibbs.html.
11. Calculations described in: Michael P. Wilson. "Green Chemistry in California: A Framework for Leadership in Chemicals Policy and Innovation." California Policy Research Center, University of California, Berkeley; March 2006 — a special report prepared for the California Senate Environmental Quality Committee and the California Assembly Committee on Environmental Safety and Toxic Materials.
12. US Centers for Disease Control and Prevention. "Chronic Disease Overview." [online]. [cited May 7, 2007]. Date last reviewed: 11/18/2005. cdc.gov/nccdphp/overview.htm.
13. S. Janssen, G. Solomon and T. Schettler. Collaborative on Health and the Environment. "CHE Toxicant and Disease Database." [online]. [cited May 7, 2007]. 2005. database.healthandenvironment.org. Also see "Collaborative on Health and the Environment Consensus Statement." [online]. [cited May 7, 2007]. healthandenvironment.org/about/consensus.
14. Theo Colborn, Dianne Dumanoski and John Peterson Meyers. *Our Stolen Future: Are We Threatening our Fertility, Intelligence and Survival? A Scientific Detective Story.* Penguin, 1997.
15. Based on 2005 update, 59.7% of personal care products analyzed in the database contained estrogenic chemicals and other endocrine disruptors. *Skin Deep.* "Summary of Major Findings." [online]. [cited May 4, 2007]. ewg.org/reports/skindeep2/findings/index.php?content=major_findings#begin.
16. Quote from Theo Colborn from public statement at 2007 UCSF-CHE Summit on Environmental Challenges to Reproductive Health and Fertility, sponsored by University of California, San Francisco and the Collaborative for Health and the Environment. See ucsf.edu/coe/prhesummit.html for information about the presentations at this historic conference. For an overview of scientific studies and discussion of the broad trends in science since the publication of *Our Stolen Future,* see ourstolenfuture.org.
17. As an example, animal studies show that bisphenol A, an estrogenic chemical found in polycarbonate baby bottles, can cause biological impacts at doses thousands of times lower than the EPA's predicted "safe dose" for humans. See Frederick S. vom Saal and Claude Hughes. "An Extensive New Literature Concerning Low-Dose Effects of Bisphenol A Shows the Need for a New Risk Assessment." *Environmental Health Perspectives,* Vol. 113, no. 8 (August 2005).
18. See Pete Myers. "Good Genes Gone Bad: The new public health reflects our understanding of how environmental contaminants damage genes." [online]. [cited April 22, 2007]. *American Prospect,* April 8, 2006. ourstolenfuture.org/newscience/lowdose/2006/2006-0401goodgenesgonebad.html.

19. As one example, the widely used pesticide Atrazine feminizes male frogs, according to researchers. When the researchers combined Atrazine with 10 other chemicals·typically applied to Nebraska corn fields, the mixture had adverse effects on the frogs that far exceed the effect of any one chemical alone. See Tyrone Hayes et al. "Pesticide mixtures, endocrine disruption, and amphibian declines: are we underestimating the impact." *Environmental Health Perspectives.* Vol. 114, No. S-1 (April 2006). [Online 24 January 2006].

20. See National Cancer Institute. "DES (Diethylstilbestrol). [online]. [cited May 5, 2007]. cancer.gov/cancertopics/des.

21. Becky Thompson. "Is Lead Inside Lipstick?" [online]. [cited May 5, 2007]. WPXI, Pittsburgh, July 24, 2006. wpxi.com/consumer/9566833/detail.html; Randy Paige. "Dangerous Levels of Lead in Lipstick, Lip Gloss?" [online]. [cited May 5, 2007]. Los Angeles affiliate CBS, May 17, 2006. cbs2.com/consumer/local_story_137185318.html.

22. As reported by WPXI, see link above.

23. E-mail sent to emma_lougener@boardermail.com on Thursday, September 9, 2004 14:27:15 -0400; subject line "Re: In response to your comments from the Revlon website, 001316821A."

24. Natasha Singer. "Should you Trust your Makeup?" *New York Times,* February 15, 2007.

25. See US Food and Drug Administration. "FDA Authority over Cosmetics." [online]. [cited May 7, 2007]. Document dated March 3, 2005. cfsan.fda.gov/~dms/cos-206.html.

26. Calculations described in Wilson (see note 11, above).

27. See safemilk.org.

## Chapter 2

1. B.C. Blount et al. "Levels of seven urinary phthalate metabolites in a human reference population." *Environmental Health Perspectives,* Vol. 108, no. 10 (October 2000), pp. 979-982.

2. The October 2000 Blount paper reported that women of childbearing age from the subgroup of 289 people had levels of DBP in their bodies up to 20 times greater than the general population. A subsequent reanalysis of the data found that women of all ages had higher levels of phthalates in their bodies than men, though not as high as originally reported. Subsequent biomonitoring studies have also found that women have higher levels of phthalates in their bodies than men. See US Centers for Disease Control. "Third National Report on Human Exposure to Environmental Chemicals." [online]. [cited April 25, 2007]. cdc.gov/exposurereport/pdf/results_06.pdf, pp. 260-261.

3. Quote by Earl Gray from lunch meeting, January 10, 2006, before two California legislative committees heard debate about Assembly Bill 319, introduced by Assemblywoman Wilma Chan (D-Alameda). The bill would have prohibited baby toys and feeding products from containing phthalates and bisphenol A.

4. National Toxicology Program, US Department of Health and Human Services, Center for the Evaluation of Risks to Human Reproduction. "NTP-CERHR Expert Panel Report on Di(2-ethylhexyl) Phthalate." [online]. [cited April 25, 2007]. October 2000. cerhr.niehs.nih.gov/chemicals/dehp/DEHP-final.pdf.

5. Jane Houlihan and Richard Wiles. *Beauty Secrets: Does a Common Chemical in Nail Polish Pose Risks to Human Health?* Environmental Working Group, November 2000.

6. Ibid, p. 3.

7. Full test results are available in: Jane Houlihan, Charlotte Brody and Bryony Schwan. *Not Too Pretty: Phthalates, Beauty Products and the FDA.* [online]. [cited April 25, 2007]. Environmental Working Group, Coming Clean and Health Care Without Harm, July 8, 2002. safecosmetics.org/docUploads/NotTooPretty_r51.pdf.

8. Ibid.

9. Joseph DiGangi, PhD. and Helena Norin. *Pretty Nasty: Phthalates in European Cosmetic Products.* Health Care Without Harm, Swedish Society for Nature Conservation, Women's Environmental Network, November 2002.

10. Seventh amendment to Council Directive 76/768/EEC on the approximation of the laws of the Member States relating to cosmetics products. See "Directive 2003/15/EC of the European Parliament and of the Council of 27 February 2003." [online]. [cited May 7, 2007]. safecosmetics.org/docUploads/DIRECTIVE%202003%5F15%5FEC%2Epdf.

11. Pat Phibbs. "Chemical Safety: Significant Effect on Cosmetics Makers Possible if EU Bans Chemicals as Proposed." *Chemical Regulation Reporter,* Vol. 26, no. 47, December 2, 2002.

12. Shanna H. Swan et al. "Decrease in Anogenital Distance among Male Infants with Prenatal Phthalate Exposure." *Environmental Health Perspectives,* Vol. 113, no. 8 (August 2005).

13. Marian Stanley quoted in: Peter Waldman. "Ingredient in cosmetics, toys a safety concern." *Wall Street Journal,* October 04, 2005. This article provides an excellent overview of the emerging data on phthalates.

14. Russ Hauser et al. "Altered Semen Quality in Relation to Urinary Concentrations of Phthalate Monoester and Oxidative Metabolites." *Epidemiology,* Vol. 17, no. 6, November 2006.

15. Russ Hauser et al. "DNA damage in human sperm is related to urinary levels of phthalate monoester and oxidative metabolites." *Human Reproductive Advance Access,* dio:10.1093/humrep/del428. Also see Dr. Hauser's and Susan Duty's first study on the DNA damage in sperm as it relates to the phthalate DEP: Susan M. Duty et al. "The Relationship between Environmental Exposure to Phthalates and DNA Damage in Human Sperm Using the Neutral Comet Assay." [online]. [cited April 25, 2007]. *Environmental Health Perspectives,* Vol. 111, no. 9 (July 2003). ehponline.org/docs/2003/5756/abstract.pdf.

16. Susan M. Duty, Robin M. Ackerman, Antonia M. Calafat and Russ Hauser. "Personal Care Product Use Predicts Urinary Concentrations of Some Phthalate Monoesters." *Environmental Health Perspectives,* Vol. 113, no. 11 (November 2005), pp. 1530—1535. Published online July 18, 2005. doi: 10.1289/ehp.8083.

17. From Shanna Swan testimony, January 10, 2006, before two California legislative committees heard debate about Assembly Bill 319, introduced by Assemblywoman Wilma Chan (D-Alameda). The bill (see note 3) died in committee but was reintroduced in 2007.

18. Shanna Swan. "Parents needn't wait for legislation to shield kids from toxins in products." *San Francisco Chronicle* op ed, January 9, 2006.

## Chapter 3

1. Jane Houlihan with Richard Wiles, Kris Thayer and Sean Gray. *Body Burden: The Pollution in People.* Environmental Working Group, January 2003.
2. The ad with Andrea Martin's story ran in the *New York Times* in January 2003.
3. Andrea Martin quotes are from a press conference at the Environmental Working Group offices in Washington DC, January 2003. See: Stacy Malkan. "Pollution of the People." [online]. [cited April 26, 2007]. Alternet, May 8, 2003. alternet.org/envirohealth/15856/.
4. From notes taken by Bryony Schwan, based on telephone conversations with Tim Long on March 3, March 5 and March 12, 2003. Conference call with representatives of campaign for safe cosmetics took place March 12.
5. Letter from Estée Lauder Inc. dated March 30, 2004, signed by Adair D. Sampogna, Vice President Global Consumer Communications, the Estée Lauder Companies Inc.
6. Statement on letterhead of the Cosmetic, Toiletry, and Fragrance Association dated March 25, 2004, entitled "CTFA Response Statement Breast Cancer Fund Letter."
7. Letter by Gap Inc., April 30, 2004, Elizabeth Muller, Environmental Manager.
8. Letter by Coty Inc., May 3, 2004, Bernd Beetz, Chief Executive Officer.
9. Letter by Custom Esthetics Ltd., April 21, 2004, Catherine M. Young, Director of Operations.
10. Letter by Blistex Inc., May 3, 2004, M.J. Donnantuono, President.
11. The ad, designed by Fenton Communications, ran in the *Washington Post* November 19, 2002.
12. E-mail from Lee Hunter at Unilever.com addressed to Maryanne Dixon, dated September 1, 2004; tracking #5768884.
13. E-mail from Consumer Affairs CKCC at Unilever.com addressed to K. Stanston, dated September 14, 2004.
14. Eui-Sun Yoo, PhD, et al. "Phthalates in Cosmetics in Korea." Citizens' Institute for Environmental Studies and Seoul Branch of the Korean Federation for Environmental Movement, April 2003.
15. Letter from Unilever Korea dated July 31, 2003, addressed to Women's Committee, Seoul Branch of the Korean Federation for Environmental Movement (KFEM), signed by Tae-Hyun Chang, Director of the Central Research Center, Unilever Korea; Ref. No.: ULK-Development-03-0731A.
16. Letter on Procter & Gamble letterhead, Newcastle-upon-Tyne offices, dated January 15, 2003, addressed to Ms. Helen Lynn, Women's Environmental Network; signed by Kathy Rogerson, P&G Beauty Technical External Relations.
17. Thaddeus Herrick. "Amid Health Concerns, Nail-Polish Makers Switch Formulas." *Wall Street Journal*, April 19, 2004.
18. Letter from Paul Hastings, Janofsky & Walker LLP, dated July 15, 2004, signed by Robert Sherman; addressed to Ms. Janet Nudelman, Director of Programs, the Breast Cancer Fund.

19. Letter from Jeanne Rizzo, Executive Director, the Breast Cancer Fund, dated September 2, 2004; addressed to Lindsay Owen-Jones, Chief Executive Officer, L'Oréal Paris.

20. The ad, designed by SmartMeme Collective, appeared in *USA Today*, New York edition in September 2005.

21. Session notes were taken by Susan Roll, assistant executive director, Massachusetts Breast Cancer Coalition at the "US and International Issues Affecting Cosmetics and OTC Drugs" session on Wednesday, September 29, 2005, from 9:00 - 12:00.

## Chapter 4

1. Cosmetic, Toiletry, and Fragrance Association. *CIR Compendium*. Published annually and available from ctfa-bookstore.org.

2. Environmental Working Group. *Farm Subsidy Database*. [online]. [cited March 28, 2007]. ewg.org/farming.

3. Environmental Working Group. *Skin Deep*. [online]. [cited March 28, 2007]. ewg.org/reports/skindeep/. The report was first published in June 2004, updated in October 2005, with a new update slated for summer 2007. *Skin Deep* data in this chapter are based on the 2005 update. The 2007 update is available at CosmeticDatabase.com.

4. Citizen petition to US Food and Drug Administration submitted by Environmental Working Group requesting cessation of unlawful sale of misbranded and adulterated cosmetics; Exhibit B (products containing ingredients that may cause harm when used according to package directions). [online]. [cited April 26, 2007]. Petition filed June 14, 2004. cosmeticsdatabase.com/research/fdapetition.php cosmeticsdatabase.com/research/impurities.php

5. Environmental Working Group. *Skin Deep*, "Summary of Major Findings." [online]. [cited March 28, 2007]. Based on 2005 update. ewg.org/reports/skindeep2/findings/index.php?content=major_findings#begin.

6. David Steinman. *Safe Trip to Eden: Ten Steps to Save Planet Earth from the Global Warming Meltdown*. Thunder's Mouth, 2006.

7. Ibid., pp. 93-136.

8. Campaign for Safe Cosmetics. "Cancer-Causing Chemical Found in Children's Bath Products." [online]. [cited April 26, 2007]. Press release, February 7, 2007. safecosmetics.org/newsroom/press.cfm?pressReleaseID=21.

9. For more information about 1,4-dioxane in personal care products see: Campaign for Safe Cosmetics. "Frequently Asked Questions about 1,4-Dioxane." [online]. [cited July 11, 2007]. safecosmetics.org/faqs/dioxane.cfm; Environmental Working Group. "EWG Research Shows 22 Percent of All Cosmetics May Be Contaminated With Cancer-Causing Impurity." [online]. [cited April 27, 2007]. Press release, February 8, 2007. ewg.org/node/21286.

10. The statistic that one in every five adults is potentially exposed every day to all of the top seven carcinogenic impurities is based on an analysis of FDA and industry reports compiled in *Skin Deep*, and an online survey conducted by EWG in 2004 of cosmetics and personal care products used by 2,300 people. See ewg.org/node/21286.

11. David Steinman and Samuel Epstein, MD *Safe Shopper's Bible: A Consumer's Guide to Nontoxic Household Products, Cosmetics, and Food.* Wiley Publishing, 1995; also Environmental Working Group. "Impurities of Concern in Personal Care Products." [online]. [cited March 28, 2007]. ewg.org/reports/skindeep2/impurities.php.

12. Advanced search function can be found at CosmeticDatabase.com/search.php.

13. Environmental Working Group. *Skin Deep.* "Summary of Major Findings." [online]. [cited March 28, 2007]. ewg.org/reports/skindeep2/findings/index.php?content=major_findings#begin.

14. A.C. de Groot and P.J. Frosch. "Adverse reactions to fragrances. A clinical review." [online]. [cited April 30, 2007]. *Contact Dermatitis,* Vol. 36, no. 2 (February 1997), pp. 57-86. ncbi.nlm.nih.gov/entrez/query.fcgi?cmd=Retrieve&db=PubMed&list_uids= 9062742&dopt=Abstract; also T. Jansson and M. Loden. "Strategy to decrease the risk of adverse effects of fragrance ingredients in cosmetic products." *American Journal of Contact Dermatitis,* Vol. 12, no. 3 (2001), pp. 166-9.

15. Consumer Reports ShopSmart. "What you should know about chemicals in your cosmetics." January 2007.

16. Jane Houlihan, Charlotte Brody, and Bryony Schwan. *Not Too Pretty: Phthalates, Beauty Products and the FDA.* Environmental Working Group, Health Care Without Harm and Coming Clean, July 8, 2002, p. 1.

17. EU's Scientific Committee on Cosmetic Products and Non-food Products. "Opinion Concerning Fragrance Allergies in Consumers: A review of the problem; analysis of need for appropriate consumer information and identification of consumer allergies." Adopted by SCCNFP during plenary session of December 8, 1999.

18. Committee on Science and Technology. "Neurotoxins: At Home and the Workplace." Report submitted to US House of Representatives, June 1986; also based on testimony from Subcommittee on Investigations and Oversight hearings to examine the subject of neurotoxins, October 8 and 9, 1985.

19. Petition 99P-1340 was filed with the FDA in 1999 by the Environmental Health Network of California. It asks that the FDA enforce existing labeling laws so consumers can make informed choices. For more information, see fpinva.org/petition99P1340.htm.

20. Alexandra Gorman and Philip O'Conner. *Glossed Over: Health Hazards Associated with Toxic Exposure in Nail Salons.* [online]. [cited April 6, 2007]. Women's Voices for the Earth, 2007. womenandenvironment.org/newsreports/issuereports/WVE.NailSalon.Report.pdf.

21. *NAILS Magazine* (2006), August 28, 2006. The NAILS Magazine 2005-2006 Big Book available for purchase at nailsmag.com/resources/industrystats.aspx.

22. C. Roelofs et al. "Nail Salons: Health Effects and Work Environment Characteristics." [online]. [cited April 27, 2007]. Presented at the American Industrial Hygiene Conference, Chicago, IL, May 17, 2006. aiha.org/aihce06/handouts/po125roelofs.pdf.

23. National Asian Pacific American Women's Forum. "The Nail Salon Industry: The Impact of Environmental Toxins on API Women's Reproductive Health." [online]. [cited April 27, 2007]. May 2006 napawf.org/file/issues/issues-Nail_Salon.pdf.

24. Environmental Working Group. "Citizen petition to cease unlawful sale of misbranded and adulterated cosmetics." FDA response denying the petition is described at: EWG. "Consumer Update — FDA admits inability to ensure the safety of personal care products." [online]. [cited July 11, 2007]. October 5, 2005. CosmeticDatabase.com/research/fdafails.php.

25. G. Oberdorster. "Manufactured nanomaterials (fullerenes, C60) induce oxidative stress in the brain of juvenile largemouth bass." *Environmental Health Perspectives,* Vol. 112 (2004), pp. 1058-1062; G. Oberdorster et al. "Nanotoxicology: an emerging discipline from studies of ultrafine particles." *Environmental Health Perspectives,* Vol. 113, no. 7 (2005), pp. 823-839.

26. Ibid.

27. Friends of the Earth. "Nanomaterials, sunscreens and cosmetics: Small Ingredients Big Risks." [online]. [cited March 28, 2007]. May 2006. foe.org/camps/comm/nanotech/nanocosmetics.pdf.

28. Keay Davidson. "FDA urged to limit nanoparticle use in cosmetics and sunscreens." *San Francisco Chronicle.* May 17, 2006.

## Chapter 5

1. SK-II website. [online]. [cited April 22, 2007]. sk2us.com/index.htm.

2. "Furious women protest in Shanghai over flawed US-Japanese cosmetics." *Agence France Presse,* September 21, 2006.

3. Matthew Evans, Ellen Groves and Michelle Edgar. "P&G Suspends SK-II Sales in China." *Women's Wear Daily,* September 25, 2006. Also see "Consumers angry as SK-II pulled off shelves." *China Daily,* September 23, 2006.

4. Cliff Peale. "P&G to resume sales in China." *Cincinnati Enquirer,* October 25, 2006.

5. Environmental Working Group. *Skin Deep.* Product search for Physicians Complex 6% Skin Bleaching Cream owned by CosMed. [online]. [cited April 22, 2007].

6. "SK-II Gets Under Consumers' Skin." *People's Daily Online.* [online]. [cited April 4, 2007]. September 25, 2006. english.people.com.cn/200609/25/eng20060925_306136.html.

7. Radio interview with Dr. Christopher Lam. "ASIA: Whitening cream sales soar as Western suntans shunned." [online]. [cited April 4, 2007]. Radio Australia, January 4, 2004. abc.net.au/ra/asiapac/programs/s1079323.htm; and "Experts Warn of Dangers of 'Skin Whitener' Creams." Reuters News service, September 26, 2006.

8. Claire Briney. "Asia-Pacific skin care: high margins fuel sales." [online]. [cited April 5, 2007]. *Euromonitor,* June 24, 2002. euromonitor.com/Asia-Pacific_skin_care_high_margins_fuel_sales.

9. Jiang Wei. "Face Value." [online]. [cited April 5, 2007]. *China Daily,* November 20, 2006. chinadaily.com.cn/bw/2006-11/20/content_737094.htm.

10. *Wet Dreams and False Images.* Jesse E. Epstein Director, 12 min. New Day Films. [DVD]. newday.com/films/WetDreams.html.

11. See Chapter 6 for more information.

12. Statistics on ethnic beauty product use from MRI Buying Styles Fall 2005; Roper NOP World Health and Beauty Aids Study May 2005; Yankelovich Monitor

Multicultural Marketing Study 2005 (in collaboration with Burrell and Karzenny/FSU), as reported on Essence.com.

13. Based on a search of *Skin Deep* 2006, a custom safety assessment of 19 products chosen with the "personal favorites" search function.

14. Mallinckrodt Baker, Inc. "Triethanolamine Material Safety Data Sheet." [online]. [cited April 4, 2007]. jtbaker.com/msds/englishhtml/t5291.htm.

15. Lewis Carroll. *Alice's Adventures in Wonderland*. MacMillan, 1938, p. 11.

## Chapter 6

1. R.G. Ziegler et al. "Migration patterns and breast cancer risk in Asian American women." *Journal of the National Cancer Institute*, Vol. 85, no. 22 (1993), pp. 1819-27.

2. Nancy Evans, ed. *State of the Evidence 2006: What is the Connection Between the Environment and Breast Cancer?* 4th ed. Breast Cancer Fund, 2006. Available from breastcancerfund.org/evidence.

3. Sandra Steingraber. "The Falling Age of Puberty in US Girls: What We Know, What We Need to Know." Breast Cancer Fund, March 2007.

4. Julia Green Brody et al. "2007. *Cancer*, 109 (S11): 2429-2473. [online]. [May 14, 2007, print June 15, 2007]. Also see the searchable online database of mammary carcinogens at sciencereview.silentspring.org/index.cfm [online]. [cited May 22, 2007].

5. Skeptics contend that synthetic estrogens are much weaker than the body's own estrogen; but unlike a woman's own estrogen, synthetic varieties are not as easily metabolized or excreted — some can linger in the body for decades. Exposures to various estrogenic substances can also add up, and they may have a much more potent effect on a fetus, small child or teenager whose breasts are developing. Evidence shows that early-life exposures to synthetic estrogens may set girls up for developing breast cancer later in life. An example is the pharmaceutical drug DES (see Chapter 1). *State of the Evidence 2006* lists several studies linking estrogenic exposures during critical windows of development to higher risk of breast cancer.

6. P.M. Ravdin et al. "The decrease in breast-cancer incidence in 2003 in the United States." *New England Journal of Medicine*, Vol. 356, no. 16 (April 19, 2007), pp. 1670-1674.

7. J.Y. Song et al. "Time Trends in Invasive Breast Cancer in the U.S. Seer System: Reporting Delay-Adjusted Increases in Invasive Breast Cancer in the U.S. SEER System 1975-2003." Abstract #132650, Presented at American Public Health Association, Boston, Mass., November 7, 2006.

8. M. Donovan et al. "Personal care products that contain estrogens or xenoestrogens may increase breast cancer risk." *Medical Hypotheses*, Vol. 68, no. 4 (2007), pp. 756- 766.

9. Reported by Anita Srikameswaran. "Care products may put black women at higher risk to develop breast cancer." *Pittsburgh Post-Gazette*, November 8, 2006. Subsequent quotes from Devra Davis in this chapter are from a personal interview in December 2006.

10. Evans, *State of the Evidence*, p. 50.

11. Breast Cancer Action. "Critical Questions to Ask." [online]. [cited April 5, 2007]. Think Before You Pink website. thinkbeforeyoupink.org/Pages/CriticalQuestions.html.

12. "Top 20 Brands of Concern." [online]. [cited April 5, 2007]. *Skin Deep* report version 2, updated October 5, 2005. ewg.org/reports/skindeep2/findings/index.php?content=brands_of_concern#begin.

13. Product listing from brand name search for products made by Avon, Estée Lauder and Revlon. [online.]. [cited April 5, 2007]. *Skin Deep* database. ewg.org/reports/skindeep/.

14. Revlon, Avon and Estée Lauder are all members of CTFA (ctfa.org/Content/NavigationMenu/About_CTFA/Member_Company_List/Active_Members1/Active_MembersJKL.htm#L). The US state of California recorded lobby efforts by CTFA at cal-access.ss.ca.gov/Lobbying/Employers/Detail.aspx?id=1143074&session=2005&view=activity). Procter & Gamble (cal-access.ss.ca.gov/Lobbying/Employers/Detail.aspx?id=1143074&session=2005&view=activity) and Estée Lauder, Inc. (cal-access.ss.ca.gov/Lobbying/Employers/Detail.aspx?id=1143074&session=2005&view=activity) are in addition individually registered as lobbyists in California.

15. Barbara Ehrenreich. "Welcome to Cancerland: A Mammogram Leads to a Cult of Pink Kitsch." Harper's, November 2001.

16. Reported by Sandy Fernandez. "Pretty in Pink." *MAMM* magazine, June/July 1998. See thinkbeforeyoupink.org/Pages/PrettyInPink.html.

17. Lisa Belkin. "Charity Begins at ... the Marketing Meeting, the Gala Event, the Product Tie-In" *New York Times,* December 22, 1996.

18. Ehrenreich, "Welcome to Cancerland."

19. Fernandez, "Pretty in Pink."

20. Ibid.

21. Sharon Batt and Liza Gross. "Cancer, Inc." *Sierra,* September/October 1999. Available online at sierraclub.org/sierra/199909/cancer.asp.

22. Monte Paulsen. "The cancer business: The same companies that profit from breast cancer treatments also manufacture." *Mother Jones,* May/June 1994.

23. Batt and Gross, "Cancer, Inc."

24. Lauren Naversen Geraghty. "Should You Worry About the Chemicals in Your Makeup?" *New York Times,* July 7, 2005.

25. National Toxicology Program, US Department of Health and Human Services, Center for the Evaluation of Risks to Human Reproduction. "NTP-CERHR Monograph on the Potential of Human Reproductive and Developmental Effects of Di(2-Ethylhexyl) Phthalate (DEHP)." November 2006. Available online at cerhr.niehs.nih.gov/chemicals/dehp/DEHP-Monograph.pdf. In its 2006 review, the NTP agreed with a 2001 NTP expert panel that DEHP poses a risk to human development and reproduction. Animal testing considered by scientists to be relevant to humans shows that DEHP can cause testicular damage, reduced fertility, abnormal sperm counts, miscarriage and birth defects.

26. See the website at lookgoodfeelbetter.org.

27. The website of "Look Good...Feel Better for Teens" is 2bme.org/2bMe.html.

## Chapter 7

1. Breast cancer rates in Marin County rose 60% between 1991 and 1999, as compared to increases of less than 5% in other areas. Breast cancer rates for white women aged 45-64 in Marin County are 58% higher than in other parts of the Bay Area (Northern California) and 72% higher than in other urban parts of California. See: Northern California Cancer Center. "Frequently Asked Questions about Breast Cancer in Marin County." [online]. [cited April 6, 2007]. co.marin.ca.us/depts/BS/main/sups/sdistr4/docs/FAQ_breast_cancer_in_Marin.pdf.
2. The cancer rate mapping project is ongoing. For more information about the Marin Cancer Project, see searchforthecause.org.
3. Marjie Lundstrom. "Powder flies as backers, foes press positions on cosmetics bill." *Sacramento Bee,* September 29, 2005.
4. CalAccess. "Lobbying Activity." [online]. [cited April 21, 2007]. cal-access.ss.ca.gov/Lobbying/. Based on a review of state records of lobbying money spent by Procter & Gamble and CTFA in California in 2005, in quarters listing SB 484 under "bills/agencies lobbied." This does not include money spent by other individual cosmetic manufacturers on SB 484.
5. Jessica Assaf. "Lobbying." [online]. [cited April 21, 2007]. Teen Ink website. teenink.com/Past/2007/February/21022.html.
6. Lundstrom, "Powder flies ..."
7. The ad, created by the SmartMeme Collective, commissioned by the Campaign for Safe Cosmetics, ran in *USA Today,* New York edition in September 2006.
8. The descriptions which follow are based on notes ("HBA September 2005 Session Notes — CTFA Regulatory Affairs: US and International Issues Affecting Cosmetics and OTC Drugs") taken by Susan Roll, assistant executive director of the Massachusetts Breast Cancer Coalition and member of the Campaign for Safe Cosmetics at the 2005 Health and Beauty America conference in September 2005.
9. Dibutyl phthalate, toluene and formaldehyde are on California's Proposition 65 list of chemicals known to the state to cause cancer or reproductive toxicity. Dibutyl phthalate is banned in the European Union because of its designation as a highly suspected reproductive toxicant. Toluene and formaldehyde are listed by the US National Toxicology Program as "reasonably anticipated" to be human carcinogens.
10. From Felicia Eaves' notes on the phone meeting with Eric Schwartz which took place on February 9, 2006.
11. The in-person meeting with Eric Schwartz took place March 30, 2006, at OPI headquarters in Los Angeles. Letters between Women's Voices for the Earth and Eric Schwartz of OPI are posted at womenandenvironment.org/campaignsandprograms/CAMPAIGN%20FOR%20SAFE%20COSMETICS/index_html.
12. Created by the SmartMeme Collective, the "OPI Miss Treatment" ad ran in the *Los Angeles Weekly* and *Variety* the week of June 27, 2006.
13. Campaign for Safe Cosmetics. "Activists and Consumers Convince OPI to Polish its Act." [online]. [cited April 21, 2007]. safecosmetics.org/companies/opi.cfm.

14. LaMont Jones. "Cosmetics makers under fire on nail polish chemicals." *Pittsburgh Post-Gazette,* Tuesday, July 18, 2006.
15. Campaign for Safe Cosmetics. "Nail Polishes to Become a Little Safer." [online]. [cited April 6, 2007]. August 30, 2006. safecosmetics.org/newsroom/press.cfm?pressReleaseID=19.

## Chapter 8

1. This and subsequent quotations are taken from the speech delivered by CTFA President & CEO Pamela G. Bailey at the CTFA 2006 Annual Meeting. A video of the speech was posted on the CTFA website: eservices.ctfa.org/Bailey_Speech.mov.
2. Dezio is the former lead spokesperson for the American Beverage Association, where she promoted soft drink vending machines in schools amidst the growing obesity crisis and defended the industry during a controversy over the discovery of benzene, a human carcinogen, in some soft drinks. See Michael Blanding. "Hard Times for Soft Drinks." [online]. [cited April 7, 2007]. *The Cold Type Reader,* May 2005, p. 6. coldtype.net/Assets.06/Essays.06/0506.Reader5.pdf.
3. Comments from Lexie Schultz are based on notes she took during the session and a subsequent personal interview in June 2006. Parts of the story also come from reporting in: Diane Farsetta. "Cosmetic Solutions: The Makeup Industry Gives Itself a Health Hazard Makeover." [online]. [cited April 22, 2007]. *PR Watch,* July 14, 2006. prwatch.org/node/4961.
4. Statements from CTFA response statement. "Lead and Cosmetics." [online]. [cited April 7, 2007]. ctfa.org.nz/information/lead/lead.html; CTFA. "Cosmetics Containing Phthalates are Safe." [online]. [cited April 7, 2007]. Press release RSPT 05-19, May 26, 2005. ctfa.org/Template.cfm?Section=CTFA_News&template=/ContentManagement/ContentDisplay.cfm&ContentID=3274.
5. Industry statements about fighting regulation, plus Dick Edmondson quote and information about Eagleton Bill, are from CTFA. "A Centennial History of CFTA." [online]. [cited April 8, 2007]. ctfa.org/Content/NavigationMenu/About_CTFA/History/History.htm.
6. E-mail exchange between Heather Serantis, on behalf of the Campaign for Safe Cosmetics, and Thomas Eagleton via Karon Hippard, legal secretary for Thompson Coburn LLP, dated September 19, 2006. Eagleton died in March of 2007 at the age of 77.
7. David Michaels. "DOUBT Is Their Product." [online]. [cited April 22, 2007]. Scientific American, Vol. 292, no. 6 (June 2005). powerlinefacts.com/Sciam_article_on_lobbying.htm.
8. Rahul Kanakia. "Tobacco Companies Obstructed Science, history professor says." [online]. [cited April 22, 2007]. EurekAlert! press release, February 18, 2007. eurekalert.org/pub_releases/2007-02/su-tco021307.php.
9. Gerald Markowitz and David Rosner. *Deceit and Denial: The Deadly Politics of Industrial Pollution.* University of California, 2002. Also see deceitanddenial.org/.

10. Gerald Markowitz and David Rosner. "'Cater to the children': The role of the lead industry in a public health tragedy, 1900-1955." [online]. [cited April 8, 2007]. *American Journal of Public Health,* Vol 90, no. 1 (2000), pp. 36-46. ajph.org/cgi/content/abstract/90/1/36.

11. Worker injuries included dissolving finger bones and angiosarcoma of the liver. For details about the internal company memos discussing industry's knowledge of the injuries, see documents posted at pbs.org/tradesecrets/program/vinyl.html.

12. Chemical Industry Archives, a project of the Environmental Working Group. "Cancer in a Can: What the Chemical Industry Kept Secret About Vinyl Chloride in Hair Spray." [online]. [cited April 8, 2007]. chemicalindustr-yarchives.org/dirtysecrets/hairspray/1.asp.

13. For a full transcript of the program, see pbs.org/tradesecrets/transcript.html.

14. Environmental Working Group. "EPA Fines Teflon Maker DuPont for Chemical Cover Up." [online]. [cited April 8, 2007]. Press release, December 14, 2005. ewg.org/issues/pfcs/20051214/index.php. This website includes a link to an archive of documents about Du Pont.

15. This ad appeared in the November 2006 issue of *Good Housekeeping* on page 45.

16 For more information about pthalates in medical devices, see NoHarm.org/US/pvcDehp/Issue. For details about the American Chemistry Council, see americanchemistry.com/essential2.

## Chapter 9

1. This and subsequent quotes are based on notes taken by Stacy Malkan at the First Annual Health and Beauty America Regulatory Summit, Jacob K. Javits Convention Center, New York City, September 13, 2006, 9:00 a.m. to 6:30 p.m. The summit was hosted by the Cosmetic, Toiletry, and Fragrance Association.

2. Ames showed several slides of decreasing deaths from cancer but not decreasing occurrence of cancer. For example, his slide for "Age adjusted cancer death rates for females in the US between 1930 and 2001" showed breast cancer death rates declining. However, the number of women who got breast cancer during that time increased dramatically.

3. One impact that REACH could have on the cosmetics industry: as more information becomes available about the toxicity of chemicals, if chemicals end up on the EU list of carcinogens, mutagens or reproductive toxicants they will be automatically banned from cosmetics.

4. Calculation based on 2006 CTFA rates Class 16 membership. Companies with $2 billion or more in cosmetics sales in 2005 must pay $395,500 plus .016% of sales over $2 billion. According to company press releases, Procter & Gamble has annual sales of $4.5 billion in just the hair care market.

5. A biological assay developed by Dr. Bruce Ames to assess the mutagenic potential of chemical compounds on bacteria. See ames-testing.com.

6. In addition to removing ingredients recognized as carcinogens or fetal toxicants in scientifically valid studies, the Compact for Safe Cosmetics asks companies to also

seek safer alternatives for chemicals recognized as endocrine disrupters, sensitizers, mutagens, reproductive toxins, developmental toxins and neurotoxins and those that are persistent in the environment and increase in concentration in the food chain.

## Chapter 10

1. Source for sales figure: "Estée Lauder Is Acquiring Maker of Natural Cosmetics." *New York Times,* November 20, 1997.
2. Jerry Adler. "The New Greening of America." *Newsweek* cover story, July 9, 2006.
3. Michael S. Rosenwald. "Showcasing the Growth of the Green Economy." *Washington Post,* October 16, 2006.
4. Consensus guidelines are being developed by the Personal Care Task Force of the Organic Trade Association; see ota.com/PersonalCareFact.html.
5. More information about German BDIH standards: kontrollierte-naturkosmetik.de/gesamt_en.htm.
6. In 2007, Avalon Organics was bought by Hains Celestial Group, the mega-corporation that owns Jason's, Zia and many other natural food and product brands. Morris Shriftman planned to stay on with the company.
7. A full list of Compact signing companies can be found at safecosmetics.org/companies/signers.cfm.

## Chapter 11

1. Janine M. Benyus. *Biomimicry: Innovation Inspired by Nature.* Harper, 2002.
2. Nanotechnology is everywhere in nature — in the form of nanostructures but not nanoparticles, which are loose, uncontrollable and unpredictable.
3. The Society of Cosmetic Chemists award for best paper was awarded to Amy S. Cannon and others for their paper, "Water Soluble Photocrosslinking Materials in Cosmetics" at the group's 2006 Annual Scientific Seminar.
4. US Environmental Protection Agency. "12 Principles of Green Chemistry." [online]. [cited April 11, 2007]. epa.gov/greenchemistry/pubs/principles.html.
5. William Greider. "Apollo Now." *The Nation,* January 2, 2006.
6. Marla Cone. "US rules allow the sale of products others ban: Chemical-laden goods outlawed in Europe and Japan are permitted in the American market." *Los Angeles Times,* October 8, 2006.
7. Michael P. Wilson, Daniel A. Chia and Brynan C. Ehlers. "Green Chemistry in California: A Framework for Leadership in Chemicals Policy and Innovation." Special Report of the University of California, Berkeley, California Policy Research Center, prepared for the California Senate Environmental Quality Committee and the California Assembly Committee on Environmental Safety and Toxic Materials, March 2006.

## Chapter 12

1. Comments made at ceremony for 2004 recipients of the Goldman Environmental Prize. To view the video of the Bhopal and Rashida Bee acceptance speech, see goldmanprize.org/node/83. To learn about the International Campaign for Justice in Bhopal, see bhopal.net.

2. Alice Walker. *We Are the Ones We Have Been Waiting For: Inner Light In a Time of Darkness*. New Press, 2006.
3. Laura Landro. "Hospitals Go 'Green' to Cut Toxins, Improve Patient Environment." [online]. [cited May 9, 2007]. *Wall Street Journal*, October 4, 2006, p. D1. noharm.org/details.cfm?ID=1395&type=document.

# Index

# About the Author

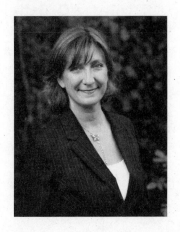

Stacy **Malkan** is Communications Director of Health Care Without Harm, and a media strategist and cofounder of the Campaign for Safe Cosmetics, an international coalition working to eliminate hazardous chemicals from personal care products. Stacy grew up in Lynn, Massachusetts, and spent several years working as a journalist and newspaper publisher in the Rocky Mountains before moving to Washington, DC, to work on environmental health campaigns. She currently lives in the San Francisco Bay Area.

For updates, visit the Toxic Beauty Blog at
www.NotJustaPrettyFace.org

If you have enjoyed *Not Just a Pretty Face* you might also enjoy other

# BOOKS TO BUILD A NEW SOCIETY

Our books provide positive solutions for people
who want to make a difference. We specialize in:

Environment and Justice • Conscientious Commerce • Sustainable Living
Ecological Design and Planning • Natural Building & Appropriate Technology
New Forestry • Educational and Parenting Resources • Nonviolence
Progressive Leadership • Resistance and Community

For a full list of NSP's titles, please call **1-800-567-6772** or check out our website at:

### www.newsociety.com

NEW SOCIETY PUBLISHERS